The Health Compass
(Plot your course to a healthy life)

Dr Beth de Sousa

Apple a Day Publishing

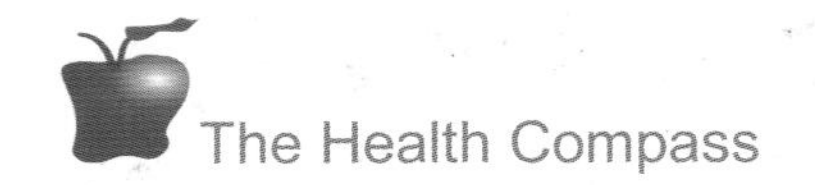

appleaday1@googlemail.com

Printed and bound by Brightsea Press

Front cover illustration by Pete Williams

ISBN 978-0-9558039

CONTENTS

Introduction

I am passionate about life and I want everyone to feel the same way.

I am a GP and I spend a lot of time talking to patients about lifestyle issues. There is a vast amount of ill health that has its root in the way we lead our lives. Don't be downhearted about this. What this means is that with the right knowledge and tools we all have the ability, within ourselves to make a meaningful and lasting difference to our own health.

There is huge potential to improve our lot with really very simple changes. Of course we are all dealt a different hand in life but what we all have is the chance to maximise our own health potential. With this book I can show you how to do this.

There have been a handful of life changing events that have led me to writing the Health Compass. Let me tell you about them.

I spent much of my teenage years and early twenties dieting. When I wasn't on a diet, I was constantly thinking about food. As a result, my weight see-sawed for many years. It wasn't until I met my lovely husband, who told me that he didn't like skinny women, that I stopped dieting and started eating regular sensible meals. My weight stabilised and to my amazement, not only was I not spending most of my day thinking about what *not* to eat, but I was the slimmest I had ever been.

Several years later, following the birth of my second child, I hurt my back badly. I spent 18 months in a cycle of pain and limitation. I took time off work and rested with little or no improvement. At the point when I thought I was never going to get better, I saw a physiotherapist who showed me how to embark on a "graded exercise programme." This system is used to add exercise in a controlled but sustainable fashion into the lives of patients. Over the next 5 years, I very gradually built a regime of exercise into my life.

I have never looked back. At 41 I feel stronger and fitter than I have ever done and wonder how I ever managed without exercise in my life.

My husband is an "ideas" person. One of the things that we laugh about is that despite having a wealth of great plans (work, home, leisure, holidays), very few of them ever get off the ground. A couple of years ago, he met a personal development coach, who showed him not only some simple techniques which both enabled him to set realistic and achievable goals but also how to incorporate them into his permanently hectic life. Following this, his life changed immeasurably. Having learnt how, he was able to make his dreams a reality.

I would like to draw a parallel between mine and my husband's situation and that of many people. If only we could be shown *how* to make changes, we could put into action all the things that we know we should be doing to improve our lives.

The UK has one of the best health care systems in the world. Despite this, as a nation, we are really not very healthy. There is an epidemic of poor health in this country and in much of the Western world, which is gathering real momentum, based largely on obesity, alcohol excess and smoking related illnesses.

Many of us have grown up with poor patterns of diet and exercise. When a pattern has been in place for a long time it can be really hard to break. This is especially true when many of our family and friends have adopted the same lifestyle. As we try to break out of the pattern, unless those around us make the same changes, we can feel isolated and find it hard to sustain the change. In addition when a habit has been in place for a long time, it can be really hard to remember what is the right thing to do.

Even those who have a good knowledge of what constitutes a healthy lifestyle, often don't know *how* to put that information into action. This can be for a variety of reasons, including time, tiredness, child care, cost, will power, motivation, or a medical problem or disability. The result is a frustrated person, who makes several attempts at change, but never seems to make any real headway.

There is a huge amount of information in the media, which focuses on these issues, but I have been frustrated by the lack of a single source which pulls all of this information together under one umbrella. After all, these areas are inextricably linked; when my patients want to lose weight, my advice is that not only should they look at what they eat and drink, but also they should be exercising more. When patients want to stop smoking, I advise them that they need to watch what they eat, or they will run the risk of putting on weight. For patients who are interested in exercising more effectively, I tell them to look at what they are eating and drinking as a way of improving their health and their performance.

I believe that we should all have equal access to a healthy lifestyle. The journey by which we achieve this is not always obvious. I therefore decided to write a guide to help you find your way. I have covered all of the main areas needed to achieve this in one book, so that you have consistent information from a single source.

I can provide you with the toolkit, with which you prepare yourself and your family, for life changes; and put those changes into action in a way that you can maintain permanently.

The changes in your diet and lifestyle should be made gently. They can be built upon over time. This could be months or even years. These changes should be realistic and manageable within your working/busy day and should therefore be maintainable for life.

Achievement is wonderful. I am regularly asked if I can prescribe a "tonic." Achievement is free of cost and side effects. For each success you will feel your self confidence grow. Confidence is infectious. Children grow up mimicking their parents in all sorts of ways. How wonderful to feel that not only could you become a role model for the way in which they lead their "health lives," but that you, as a result of positive changes that you have made in your life, could pass on some of your inner confidence to them.

Patterns set in childhood are much easier to carry into adulthood. Making a life change for not only yourself but your whole family could set a new healthier lifestyle for many future generations.

Think of looking after yourself as an investment for both you and your family's future.

Let this guide be your compass. It will help you find your way. My family and I live life by it and I hope that it can be as helpful to you as it has been to me.

Our lives and our bodies are precious. Each of us has the power to make the change

Dr Beth de Sousa

Acknowledgements

Thank you to my husband Nigel and to my children Ashe and Fynn for always being there with big hearts and open arms.

Thank you to my great buddies Stella King, Alison Troop, Monica Spanton-Coates, Jenny Caldwell, and Emily van Tinteren for their thoughts and ideas.

Karin Lake, I love that you call a spade a spade. You are Fairy Godmother to this book.

Jack Russell, Personal Development Coach and friend, without your encouragement, I would still be sitting here with a blank sheet of paper.

Tracey Beaney, my computer would be at the bottom of the fishpond, if it weren't for you.

Last of all, thank you to Karen Hall for reminding me to always cherish and to never waste a single second of life.

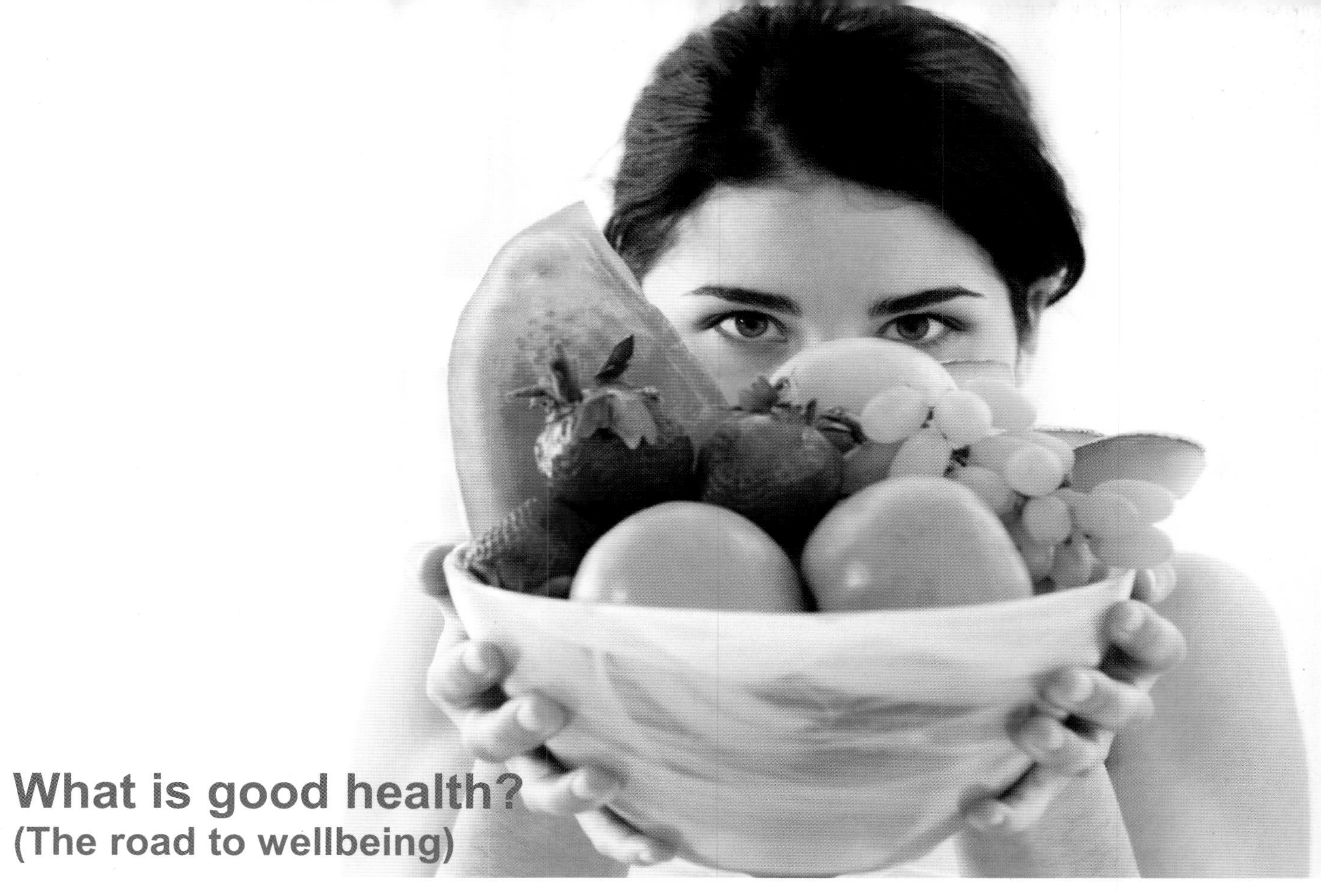

What is good health?
(The road to wellbeing)

When I ask my patients what issues are important in their lives, most people have health somewhere near the top of their list.

What does good health mean to you? Some might say, being free from a medical complaint, such as infection, heart attack, stroke or disability. For me it means all of these, plus feeling great. It is both physical and emotional wellbeing. It is about maximising enjoyment of life by giving yourself choices, because you are free of the shackles of poor health.

You don't have to have an illness or disability to suffer. If you can't walk up a flight of stairs without getting out of breath, due to obesity or smoking, you are not getting the most out of life. If you regularly can't get out of bed in the morning for work, because you have a hangover, you are not operating at 100%.

My message to you is that there are a few things you do need to know, but the basics are actually very simple and putting them into practice can be a lot of fun.

There are five main areas which I think are important to look at in order to achieve a healthy life: weight, diet, exercise, alcohol consumption and smoking. If you get it right in these areas, you will find that a whole lot more falls into place.

I will have you looking and feeling younger and fitter than you have ever felt. There is so much enjoyment to be had. The more you put into life; the more you get back. I want to show you how to make it happen. Once you get started you will wonder why you didn't do it years ago.

People will look to you as their health role model. You will glow with confidence and enthusiasm. Take a look at the next section which covers "What is good health?" and I will guide you through.

The best time to get healthy is now

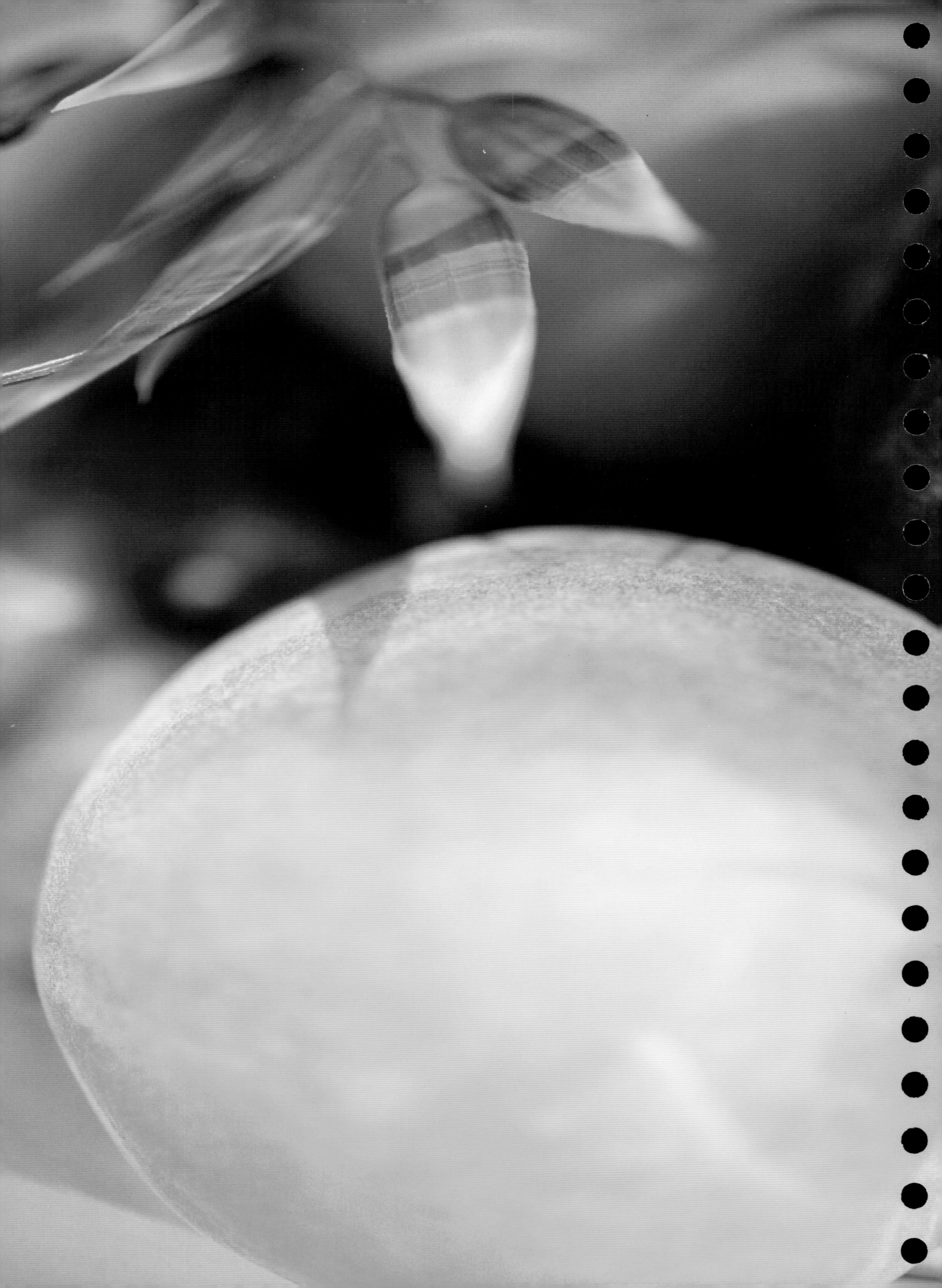

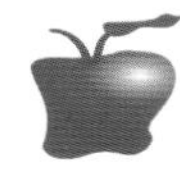

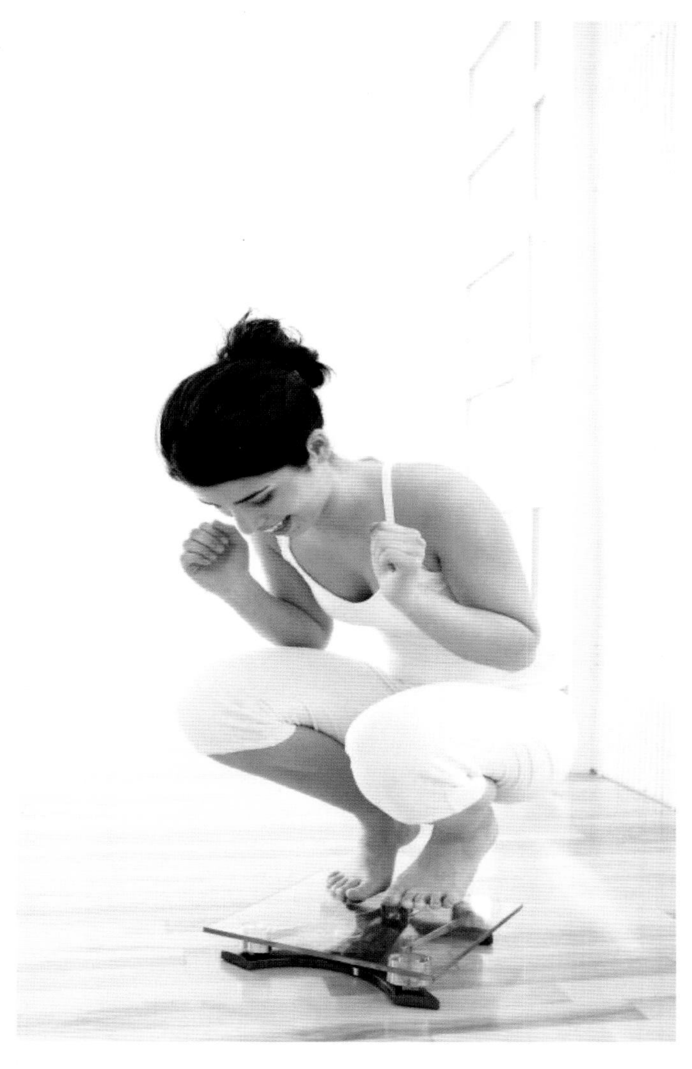

Weight
(Ditch the Bridget Jones knickers)

I play a little game when patients ask if I can weigh them. I try and guess what their weight will be before they get on the scales. A funny thing happens; more often than not I under-estimate.

Why should this be? Well either I'm really bad at guessing weight or could it be that my benchmark of what is a normal healthy weight is all wrong?

When last measured in 2005, it was found in the UK that almost two thirds of adult men and women are over weight and a quarter are obese.

In reality we see less people on the street that are a normal weight than we do of people who are not. It is easy therefore for the idea in our minds of what is healthy and what is not to be skewed.

Why is this important? In basic terms, the more overweight you are, the more likely you are to suffer with poor health.

Most people who are obese have put on weight slowly over a number of years. It is easy in these circumstances to forget what it is like to feel well.

Being overweight can have a knock on effect in many areas. It increases your risk of heart attack, stroke, high blood pressure, diabetes, breast cancer, cancer of the large bowel, gallstones, arthritis, infertility and depression.

If one of these conditions is in your family, you will prevent or delay the onset in yourself, by losing weight. If you already suffer from one of the conditions above, losing weight will help you.

I want to show you that you have the power to influence your future. Making a change to your weight could revolutionise your life. Losing weight is not about being thin, it is about instigating changes that will shape your future for the better. You will feel and look healthier and fitter and your self confidence will improve. You will have more energy and zest for life. You will be less breathless, your joints will feel freer and less painful, your indigestion will resolve, your sex life and sleep will improve and big knickers will be a thing of the past.

If you thought that you were locked into an inevitable destiny, think again. Small but sustainable changes can have a huge positive effect on your future. Forget weight loss targets as your sole aim. Make a resolution to achieve a healthy weight by healthy means. Manageable steps; one by one. I will show you how.

How do we measure weight?

OK, this is the technical bit. Stay with me, it won't last long!

Have a bit of fun and go and get your bathroom scales and a tape measure and see if you can work out your own BMI. If you don't have the energy or the inclination have a look at the website that accompanies this book on www.healthcompass.co.uk where I will calculate your BMI for you.

Health professionals use the BMI (body mass index) when measuring weight. This is a ratio which takes into account your height when measuring your weight.

If you have a BMI of between 18.5 and 24.9 your weight is in the normal range.

If your BMI is under 18.5 you are underweight.

If you have a BMI of between 25.0-29.9 you are overweight and over 30 you would be considered to be obese.

How to work out your BMI

Your weight in kg, divided by the square of your height in metres

For example a 75kg man of 1m 70cm height would have a BMI of

$$\frac{75}{1.7 \times 1.7} = 25.9$$

BMI does not take into account those who are heavy due to large muscle bulk. In addition to this, those people who carry most of their excess fat around their waistline, tend to be at a higher risk of heart disease and diabetes than others.

For this reason, we can use waist measurement as well as BMI to help.

These are the waist measurements that health professionals use to assess health risks. If your waist size is equal to or above that in the table below, you are at a higher risk of heart disease and diabetes than someone of a lower waist size.

Make sure you measure your waist in the right place, that is, half way between your lowest rib and the top of your hip bone.

Health risk	Male waist	Female waist
Increased health risk	**94cm (37 inches) or more**	**80cm (31 inches) or more**
Greatly increased health risk	**102cm (40 inches) or more**	**88cm (35 inches) or more**

Source: adapted from NICE (2006), International Diabetes Federation (2005), WHO/IASO/IOTF (2000) and World Health Organisation (2000)

Even a small sustained reduction in weight can give significant health benefits

Losing a little is a good start and is better than nothing

Losing 10kg (22lb) could mean the difference between you having to take medication for the rest of your life to control blood pressure or high cholesterol, or not. It might mean that you can stop yourself becoming diabetic and you may be able to save yourself from having a hip or knee replacement. It could prevent you developing gallstones, asthma, breast cancer, varicose veins or leg ulcers.

In other words losing weight will make you feel younger and fitter and it will keep you that way. Give yourself the freedom to enjoy life.

Don't go for bust. Think long term. Think healthy for life. Start today with a small change and keep that going. Make a note of the change you have made. It may not seem much, but if you continue over the next 10 years to add small but steady changes to your life in this way, they will accumulate and without realising, you will have not only the foundations but a sky scraper of successful change behind you.

Try this today

Choose from one of the following and keep it going:

- Cut out one of the sugars from your tea or coffee
- Swap from butter to margarine
- Reduce the number of potatoes you have on your plate by one
- Grill rather than fry your meat
- Buy semi-skimmed rather than full fat milk
- Buy standard size rather than king size chocolate bars

Myth:	You can't be fit and fat. If you don't lose weight, there's no point in exercising
Myth buster:	Overweight people who are fit have a lower risk of stroke, heart disease and diabetes than those who are not.

Why do we put on weight?

Our bodies need only a certain amount of fuel to function efficiently. Any excess is stored as fat so that in times of starvation we have a supply to tap into.

There is no doubt, some people put on weight more easily than others. Our genetics, that is the hand we were dealt with when we were born, are responsible for only 40% of our tendency to gain weight easily.

It is really easy not to bother even making a start on trying to lose weight if your parents and their parents before were heavy as there can be a sense of inevitability about your weight. This does not have to be the case. The other 60%, that is more than half, of your ability to lose weight is down to you. That is, how much and what you eat and what exercise you do.

If you eat too much or don't exercise enough, you will gain weight. The good news then, is that we all have the power to make a change.

Our diets have become saturated with ready made meals and junk food which are high in fat, sugar and salt, which is bad for your heart. This food offers a tempting quick solution if you are on a tight time schedule. It can be really hard when pushed for time, not to fall into the trap of using these foods regularly.

The offer of food is everywhere. The media floods us with images of food. Sweets, chocolate and crisps are relatively cheap and bombard you, even in places of health such as gyms and swimming pools. Often food comes in super size bags. It has become the norm to snack on chocolate and crisps which are high in calories. Is it any wonder that we struggle with our weight?

There are a few people that have hormone imbalances or who are on medication, that make it more difficult to lose weight, but these make up only 2% of the overweight population.

The most common medical condition that can cause weight gain is having an under-active thyroid. This is a small gland in your neck that secretes one of the hormones that are responsible for controlling your metabolic rate; that is how fast or slow your body goes. If your thyroid gland is under-active it can cause you to put on weight or to have trouble losing weight. However, the average weight gain from patients suffering with an under-active thyroid is only 3-5 kg (7-11 lb). If you are having trouble losing weight, it is worth checking with your doctor, who can do a blood test to rule out thyroid or other hormone imbalances.

There has been publicity recently about the "Fat Virus." Research at the University of Wisconsin has identified a virus which may be responsible for some people putting on more weight than others. In animal studies a related virus has been shown to be responsible for chickens putting on weight. At present we do not know how much weight gain the virus could be responsible for in affected individuals, if at all. Implications might be that in the future an antiviral medication or vaccine could be developed to help those people infected. It is however important that those with the virus make sure that they follow as healthy a regime as those who are not.

"Childhood is that wonderful time when all you need to do to lose weight is take a bath"

Richard Zera

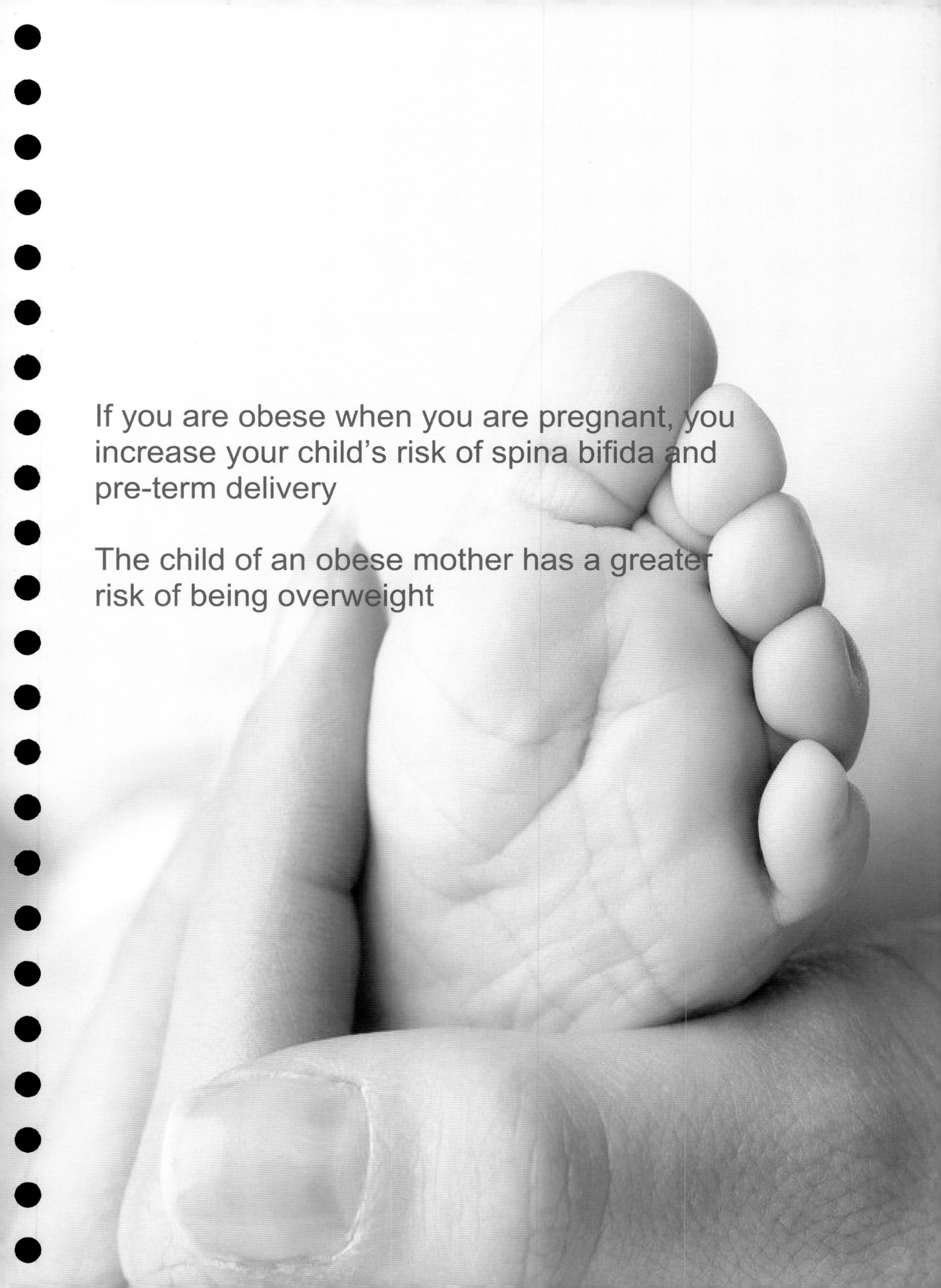

If you are obese when you are pregnant, you increase your child's risk of spina bifida and pre-term delivery

The child of an obese mother has a greater risk of being overweight

How can we lose weight?

I would really like to get away from the idea of weight loss being a continuous battle. I would also like to distance myself from the idea of "the target weight." We are all made in different shapes and sizes and some of us are blessed with more curves than others. Weight should not be an issue of clothes size or kilo counting but more about the way you feel in combination with finding the weight at which your body works best for you. You don't need a set of scales to measure that.

In order to lose weight you have to either decrease the amount of fuel you put into your body, or increase your energy expenditure. In other words we need to eat less in terms of calories or exercise more, or preferably both. There are several ways in which we can achieve this. In principle however the message is eat plentifully of the foods that help your body and go out and have some fun getting active.

The joy of eating more healthily means that unlike traditional diets which involve you cutting down your portion sizes, if you choose the right foods, you can still eat plenty. This relies on you eating smaller quantities of high calorie, nutrition free foods in exchange for eating larger quantities of lower calorie foods that are packed with goodness; foods that work with your body and benefit your health long term.

The other alternative is to eat less of foods that are high in calories in combination with cutting down your portion sizes. Most people will probably do a combination of the two.

I don't like the idea of counting calories. It is too exhausting and hard to maintain. However whichever method of weight loss you choose you do need to recognise which foods are high in calories and eat less of them.

Some examples of foods with the highest calories, both savoury and sweet are:

- Fatty foods such as fried foods, crisps, chips, roast meals, pastry, cream cheese, butter and cream
- Foods high in sugar such as sweets, chocolates, cakes, biscuits and sweet pastries

Some examples of foods which are packed with goodness and are OK to eat in abundance are:

- Fruit such as apples, kiwifruit, apricots, cranberries, grapes, oranges, lemons, limes, passion fruit, pomegranates, strawberries, peaches, nectarines, figs, bananas, pineapples, grapefruit, papaya, pears, and mangos
- Vegetables such as asparagus, parsnip, tomato, pepper, courgette, beet, broccoli, celery, cauliflower, carrot, radish and squash
- Nuts (unsalted) such as hazelnuts, almonds, brazils, pecans, walnuts, pistachios and pine nuts
- Seeds such as flax, pumpkin, sesame and sunflower
- Leafy green vegetables such as spinach, lettuce, kale, rocket, parsley, watercress, sorrel, endive and chicory
- Beans such as aduki, lentils, pinto and soybeans
- Fresh herbs such as coriander, basil, mint, parsley, sage, thyme, tarragon, fennel, rosemary, oregano, ginger, dill, bay and marjoram

Choosing foods of as wide a variety as possible should ensure that you get a broad selection of vitamins and minerals whilst maintaining an interesting and exciting diet.

Eating less high calorie foods should lead to a certain amount of weight loss, but if built into a traditional strict diet, the weight loss is often temporary, going straight back on if you resume previous eating and lifestyle habits.

There are all sorts of fad diets available to us. Some are better than others at short term weight loss. Very few people are able to maintain convincing weight loss following strict regimes because for all sorts of reasons, restrictive eating is really hard to maintain.

In addition to this, these diets may not have been tested for long term safety and may not fulfil the healthy eating requirements of a balanced diet. Fad dieters are like modern day politicians; they go for changes which are popular because they appear beneficial in the short term, while ignoring the possibility of long term harm.

Even if you don't lose weight, if you are eating a nutritious, balanced diet and exercising more, your body will be healthier. You will be protecting yourself long term from a large variety of medical problems. Just because you don't see it from the outside, doesn't mean that what's going on inside isn't good.

It is natural to crave an instant result, however if we are to maintain life changes, we need to think long term and start with the foundations, before we build the entire house. A house put up on sand is likely to fall over during the first storm.

I prefer the idea of lifestyle change, which includes dietary changes, but more along the lines of a healthy eating plan in association with an increased exercise level. This is a much more holistic way of approaching your weight management. If you need to lose weight, aim for weight loss of 0.5-1kg a week (around 1-2 lb a week). It may not lose your weight fast, but it's better to go for the long term approach. What comes off, should then stay off as long as you don't resume old unhealthy lifestyle and eating habits.

Don't aim purely to lose weight. Think in terms of healthy eating targets.

If you have a family, healthy eating is something you can do together. Unlike traditional diets it avoids isolating you from your family as you diet. You support each other. Through your children, you set a blueprint for a healthy lifestyle for future generations

If the current trend continues, children will have a shorter life expectancy than their parents, purely because of their weight

Are there any ways that we can trick our bodies into losing weight?

OK, the language is a bit tough going, but the principles are fun. Take a look, have a go and see what you think.

- Leptin is a hormone (chemical messenger) that is made by fat cells and acts as an appetite suppressant. In theory, the more fat you eat, the more leptin you produce and your appetite should be satisfied. However, the fat cells of people who are overweight, get used to the high levels of leptin and as a result, their appetites become larger, rather than smaller.

- Ghrelin is a hormone produced by the stomach that makes you feel hungry. This hormone is suppressed best by eating "good carbohydrates" such as rice, pasta, bread and potatoes and also by eating proteins such as meat, fish and pulses. It takes far more fat than carbohydrate or protein to switch off ghrelin.

So by eating less fat in your diet and replacing it with more "good" carbohydrates or proteins, you decrease your appetite.

- Leptin, the appetite suppressor is released in response to eating. Eating slowly allows time for its release. Eating fast, fills your stomach to a much greater extent, before the body has had time to tell you it's full. Therefore if you eat more slowly, you will become full having eaten less.

- Research has shown that sleep deprivation can increase Ghrelin levels (the hormone responsible for hunger). A study done at Chicago University and repeated at Bristol University (by Shahrad Taheri), with identical results shows that there is clear evidence that adult obesity has a strong connection with the amount you sleep as a child. The less you sleep, the heavier you will be as an adult. Many children have televisions in their rooms these days which has the direct effect of decreasing the amount they exercise and also runs the risk of them sleeping less. Interestingly once over the age of 16, lack of sleep has no further impact on weight.

- Exercising in the hour before a meal sets your metabolic rate at a higher level. This means that the calories you take in will be burnt off more quickly.

In summary

- Replace the fats in your diet with "good" carbohydrates and protein; it will reduce your appetite
- Eat your meals more slowly; you will feel fuller
- Make sure your children get plenty of sleep; their appetite will be smaller
- Exercise in the hour before a meal; you will burn off more calories

"Getting my lifelong weight struggle under control has come from a process of treating myself as well as I treat others in every way"

Oprah Winfrey

Are diet groups successful?

If you enjoy group activity then diet groups can be really effective. They tend to offer more traditional "diet" advice, counting calories and weighing food, but short term weight loss can be really good.

If you are to maintain your weight loss following a diet, you should not return to your original eating and exercise pattern as the weight will gradually creep back on. For this reason, while you are on your Weight Management Programme, you should make a start on adding exercise into your life. Once you have finished your programme, your exercise regime will already be established. Going back to your old dietary habits will allow the weight to go back on, possibly even if you are exercising, so it is important at this point to transfer to a healthy eating plan.

Some GP surgeries now offer Weight Management Referral Programmes. In order to be referred you may need to fulfil certain criteria, such as weighing over a certain amount, sometimes in addition to having other weight related problems, such as high blood pressure or diabetes. The different referral criteria will depend on the area in which you live, but the idea is that some patients can be referred to programmes for a reduced charge or for no charge for a fixed period of time. Check with your GP if you have one running locally.

Myth:	Restricting calorie intake is the best way to lose weight.
Myth buster:	Your metabolism slows if you severely restrict your calorie intake and so you burn less energy, which offsets the benefit of eating less.

What about medicines and surgery to reduce weight?

Your GP might consider you are suitable for help with weight loss using drug treatment if you fulfil certain criteria. You used to be required to have already lost weight before your GP would consider you for drug treatment but guidelines have recently changed and this is no longer true. If you request medication to help with weight loss, it is preferable however to show your GP that you already have a healthy lifestyle plan in place.

There are 3 drugs currently available:

- Orlistat
- Sibutramine
- Rimonabant

Orlistat

Orlistat works by blocking the gut from absorbing fat, so this is a particularly effective drug to use if you have a diet high in fat. It should not be used as a substitute for you cutting the fat out of your diet but as an aid to doing so.

Side effects of using this medication include flatulence (a lot of wind), faecal urgency (the need to urgently empty your bowels), faecal incontinence and abdominal bloating and pain. If you avoid fat, then these side effects should be minimised and this of course is a great deterrent to including fat in your diet.

Your doctor can prescribe this if :

- you have a BMI of 28 or more plus heart disease, diabetes or high cholesterol

- you have a BMI of 30 or more

In order for your doctor to continue prescribing Orlistat for you, beyond 3 months, you have to lose at least 5% of your initial body weight over the first 3 months of treatment.

The company that produce Orlistat have a support web site which gives dietary advice if you are trying to lose weight. You can only access the detailed lose weight plan if you are being prescribed the medication. Take a look on:

www.xenicalmap.co.uk

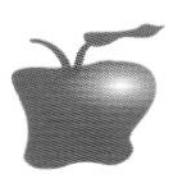

Sibutramine

This medication works by reducing your appetite. So it is particularly useful if you have a problem with reducing your portion size. Sibutramine's main side effect is that it can cause high blood pressure, so if you take this medication, your doctor will monitor your blood pressure really closely. Sibutramine should not be used in people who are currently suffering with depression as it can lead to a worsening of mood. It can however be used if you have recovered from depression as long as your doctor keeps a close eye on you.

Your doctor can prescribe this if:

- you have a BMI of 27 or more plus diabetes, heart disease, high blood pressure or high cholesterol
- you have a BMI of 30 or more

As with Orlistat, you have to demonstrate at least 5% loss of your initial body weight if you are to continue beyond 3 months of treatment and treatment is not recommended beyond 1 year.

The manufacturers of Sibutramine have a support web site with advice and support on losing weight. The beauty of this web site is that you can access it free, without being prescribed the medication. Take a look on:

www.changeforlifeonline.com

Rimonabant

This medication works by reducing appetite, by blocking appetite signals from the brain and fat that promote hunger. It is particularly useful in reducing waist size and so is good if you carry your excess weight in this area.

It can cause depression and for this reason doctors are being advised caution with prescribing until there is more safety data.

A word of warning regarding medications to aid weight loss

Most people, if using these medications in combination with a healthy eating plan will lose weight. These drugs can only be prescribed for a finite amount of time. When you stop them, unless you increase your exercise level, you will slowly regain your weight. It is therefore really important to try and establish an exercise regime of some sort while you are on them, which you continue after stopping the drugs. This will help to keep the weight off. Your exercise regime can be as little as walking for 30 minutes 5 times a week. For some fun and interesting ways of getting fit, turn to the section on exercise which begins on page 43.

Weight loss (Bariatric) surgery

Your doctor may refer you for surgery if you have had no success losing weight or your weight has reached a plateau, despite having a healthy eating and exercise plan in place. You also need to fulfil the following criteria:

- a BMI of between 35-40 in association with other obesity related illness such as diabetes or high blood pressure, that could be improved with weight loss

- a BMI of greater than 40

You do however need to be fit enough to undergo a general anaesthetic and you need to be able to commit to long term follow up, which can be quite intensive.

There are now a variety of surgical options, some of which can be via keyhole surgery (laparoscopy). This makes the operation much smaller and less risky for the patient. All areas should now be offering this on the NHS, although funding is limited at the present time. There are many private companies offering this through the internet. Make sure that if you go this route that you choose a reputable surgeon, preferably who is not too far away from you. The follow up and support are equally as important as the operation itself and if this is in a different language or too far to get to because of distance or finance, you are immediately at a disadvantage.

If you would like to check out a web site that looks at Bariatric Surgery try:

www.bospa.org or

www.patient.co.uk/showdoc/40025123

Beth's top tip:
Oats not only fill you up and help prevent sugar cravings, but are great for "soaking up" cholesterol. Eat plenty.

"If you have formed the habit of checking on every new diet that comes along, you will find that eventually, they all blur together, leaving you with only one definite piece of information: French Fries are out"

Jean Kerr

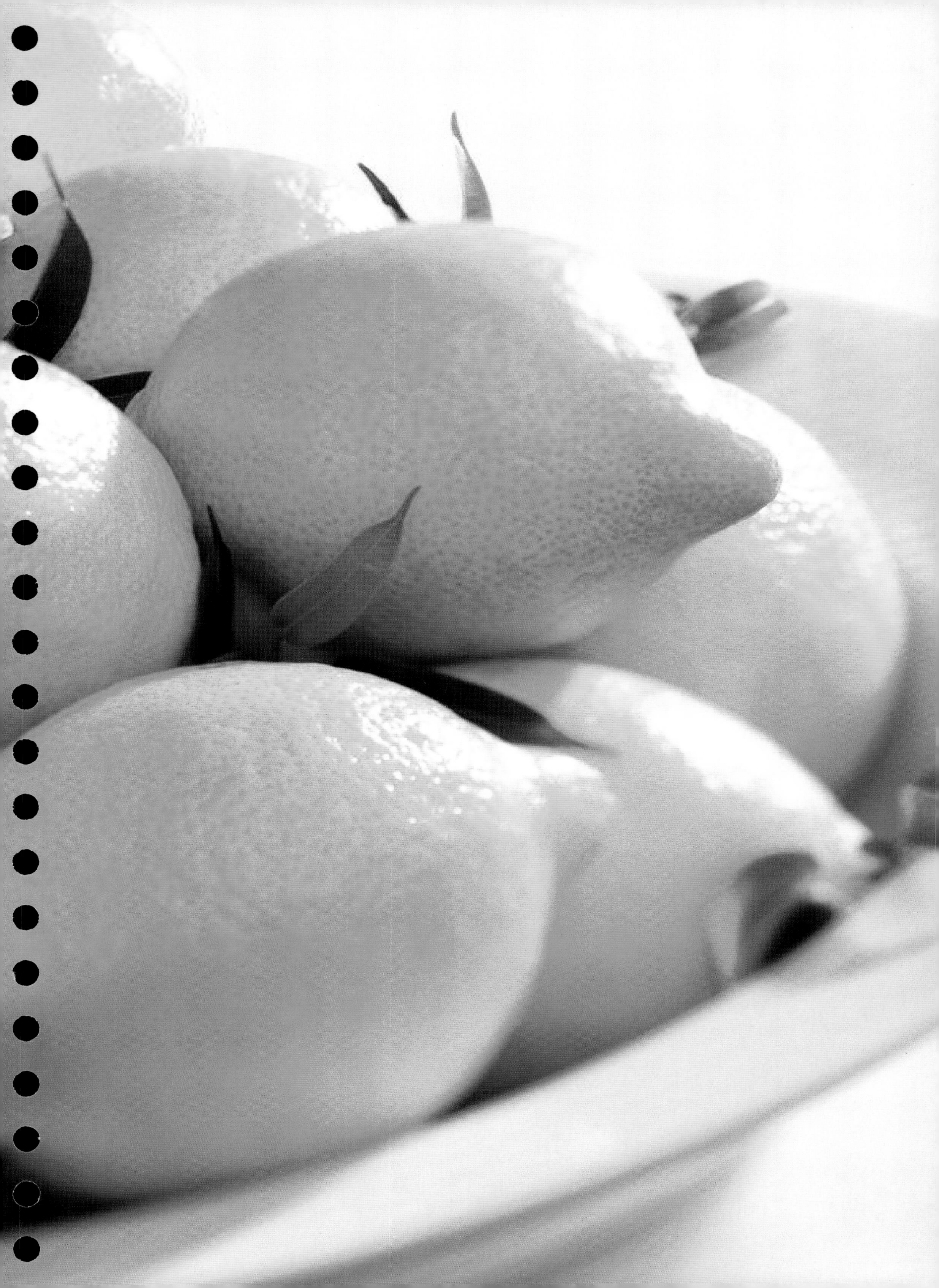

Sarah's story

Sarah is 31 years old and has just had her second baby. She plans to go back to work part time when her baby is 6 months old. Sarah gave up smoking when she discovered that she was pregnant with her first child, who is now 3 years old. She put on 10kg (1½ stone) during her first pregnancy, and never lost it. She has put on a further 5½ kg (12lb) in her second pregnancy and is now keen to lose the excess weight.

She used to do aerobics before she had children but since then has not had the time or the energy to do any exercise at all. She feels she has no life of her own. Sarah's husband works long hours, but never at the weekend.

Sarah's food diary shows the following pattern of eating:

She regularly skips breakfast and sometimes lunch. She snacks and grazes through the day, rarely sitting down to eat. Her main weaknesses are picking food off the children's plates and eating chocolate in the early evening. Sarah eats her main meal with her husband at about 8 o'clock every evening during the week when he gets in from work, by which time her appetite is poor from all the picking. She has 1-2 glasses of wine every night after the children have gone to bed to help her unwind.

Sarah's strengths are that she is good at cooking from fresh ingredients.

Having identified where she was "slipping," Sarah changed her routine. She now eats regular meals, and finds that this helps with craving for sugary things between meals. She has found that a bowl of muesli type cereal with chopped banana on it really fills her up in the mornings. She sits with the children at lunch time and eats with them, and so feels less need to snack from their plates. She does the same in the evenings during the week, to avoid the need to snack before her main meal which was previously so late. At the weekends they try to eat together earlier as a family, but sometimes she enjoys waiting until after the children have gone to bed, to eat with her husband alone.

Sarah still feels the need to snack on occasions but always keeps a bowl of fresh fruit salad in the fridge and uses this for both her and the children if she gets peckish. She also eats yoghurts as a healthy "light bite." When she gets chocolate cravings, she finds brushing her teeth really helps. When they go out, she takes a supply of cereal bars or little boxes of raisins with them in order that they are not tempted to buy crisps or chocolate as they did in the past. She still eats a couple of chocolate bars a week.

The amount of calories in a glass of wine surprised Sarah and this was a good incentive for her to try and have a couple of alcohol free days a week. She has found this really difficult to achieve, but has managed to cut down to only one glass a day, which is better than before. She does however feel much more awake on the evenings that she doesn't have a glass of wine and also finds that the sugary cravings are not so bad following an alcohol free night.

Feeling better and having lost 4kg (9lb) over the last 2 months Sarah has resolved to add exercise to her week. She has already started walking her 3 year old to pre-school and is looking forward to starting an aerobics class twice a week at her local gym, where she will be able to leave her baby in the crèche.

My thoughts

Sarah's story is obviously one of success. It is important to note however that she did not get it right first time on every occasion. This is not a criticism, but a word of encouragement to you. What we need to learn from this is that people don't always succeed on their first attempt. You are not alone. Take heart. If you stumble, pick yourself up and try again. With each attempt you will gain some ground and if you keep at it, you will get there.

How might she have gone about things differently? Well, her main concern was her weight. She gained weight initially when she stopped smoking and then during her pregnancies.

Adding exercise into your life, as you give up smoking, can be really good at preventing weight gain, rather than having to battle with it, once it's already on. Many women are shy of exercising in pregnancy, for fear of hurting the developing baby in some way. Exercise during pregnancy can be really beneficial and not only can help prevent weight gain but can reduce the length and complications of labour. Turn to the chapter on exercise for more details about how to exercise in pregnancy.

Sarah is pleased with her progress, and yet she still has some remaining goals. Notice how she doesn't tackle everything at once, but takes one area that she feels confident with, her eating habits and tackles that first. When she has established herself well in this area she moves on to the next.

She still wants to look at having one night alcohol free a week, but she chooses to shelve that until she is ready. That is the right approach for her.

Exercise is the area that she is looking at next. Establishing a routine can be difficult when you have very young children and little time. Having a helpful partner who can baby sit on a regular occasion is helpful here.

Another thing she might think about, is getting a friend to join her in an exercise class or on a brisk walk with the push-chair. This is a really good way of giving each other encouragement and support and can reduce the feeling of isolation that can occur when you have your hands full with little ones. Toddler groups and post-natal groups are a good way to meet other young mums in a similar situation.

For child care, you can look at gyms with crèches and poolside play pens. If you are lucky enough to meet a group of mums with young children, a supportive baby sitting ring can be a really good way of feeling that your baby is in good hands while you take some exercise.

Weight
(Ditch the Bridget Jones knickers)

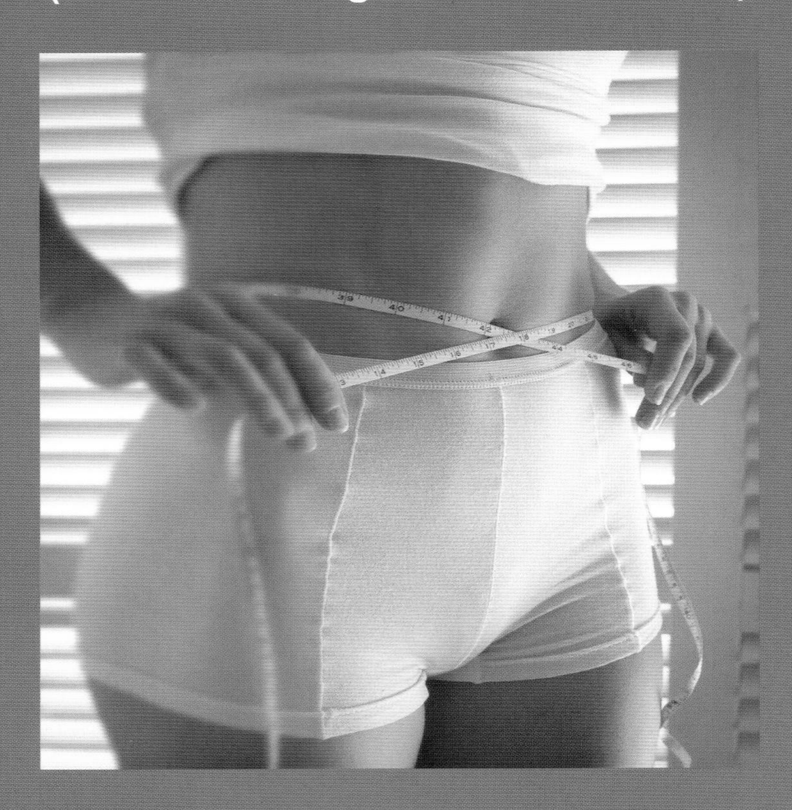

Remember

- A healthy BMI is between 18.5 and 25
- You are at extra risk of weight related health problems if you have a large waistline
- Even a small weight loss can give really big health benefits
- The best way to lose weight is to eat less and to exercise more in combination
- The ideal rate for losing weight is 0.5-1kg (1-2 lb) per week

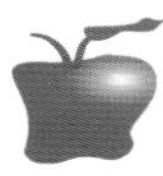

Diet
(From broad bean to runner bean)

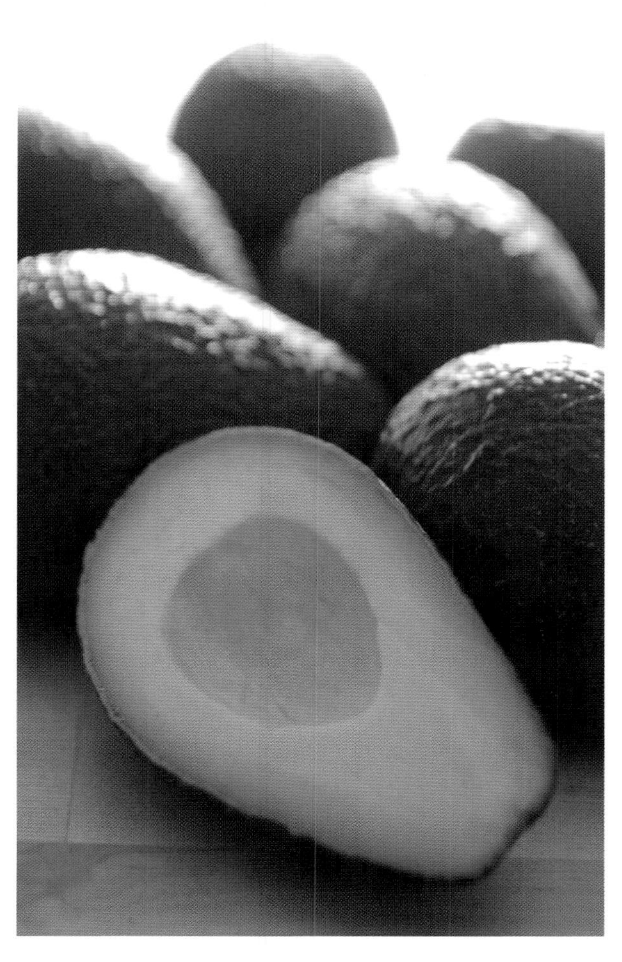

What is a healthy diet?

Eating for your health is about eating a wide variety of interesting foods that are going to work for your body and make you feel great; it's about common sense and moderation.

The message I want to get across, is that eating and living healthily is not complicated. There are a few basic facts that you need to know, but let's not get blinded by science.

Unless you have a vitamin deficiency due to a medical condition or illness, or have extra-ordinary nutritional requirements due to an intensive fitness regime, such as an elite athlete might have, you don't need to take endless dietary supplements.

There is huge focus at the moment on the way we look, fuelled by make over programmes in the media. Far more important than the way you are clothed on the outside, is the way you are clothed from within.

In order to function at maximum efficiency the body needs a balance of certain foods which will provide a combination of energy, vitamins and minerals. Get the balance and quantity right and you will feel great. You will have boundless energy, you will sleep better and you will lose weight. Your skin and hair will shine and your nails will look fantastic. Your headaches will improve as will your indigestion, joint pains, fertility and sex drive.

Small sustained changes can make a huge difference in the long term.

There are 5 food groups from which to choose. These are:

Fresh fruit and vegetables

Carbohydrates such as bread, cereals, potatoes, rice, pasta and sugary foods

Fats, such as butter, cream, fried foods and oily dressings

Proteins such as meat and fish, nuts, eggs and pulses

Dairy products, such as milk, yoghurt and cheese

What is the ideal diet?

The people of the Mediterranean have got it just right with a diet rich in fresh fish, pasta, pulses, fresh fruit and leafy green salads made with an olive oil base to the dressing. Here is a guide for you:

- Eat at least 5 portions of fresh fruit and vegetables a day. Choose from as wide a variety as possible
- Eat plenty of starchy foods such as brown bread, potatoes, rice and pasta. If you have wheat intolerance you can eat potatoes, rice, rice pasta, maize, quinoa, buckwheat, corn, millet, amaranth and tapioca as great alternative sources of slow release carbohydrate. Oats that have not been milled with wheat, barley or rye are safe and are now available in some health food shops.
- Eat moderate amounts of meat and protein. Eat less red meat as it is high in fat. Stick to white meat and fish as much as possible. Pulses, soy and tofu are a good natural source of protein containing very little fat. Nuts are higher in fat but tend to contain monounsaturated fat which can be helpful in lowering your cholesterol levels
- Eat 1 portion a week of oily fish such as mackerel, tuna, sardines or pilchards
- Eat moderate amounts of milk and dairy products but try and pick the low fat options where possible. Soya, sheep and goats milk are an easy to digest alternative
- Eat only small amounts of fatty foods. Choose low fat options if you can. Avoid ready meals, pastry, red meat or junk food, which tend to be high in fat. Grill rather than fry your food
- Replace saturated fats such as butter or lard with monounsaturated fats such as margarine and olive oil, certain nuts (see page 37) and avocados. Avoid rich sauces and dressings. Monounsaturated fats can lower your "bad" cholesterol and contain essential fats your body needs; they are good for you in moderation
- Drink plenty to flush out your kidneys and to keep your mind active. Try to drink 6-8 cups of fluid a day if possible. Filtered water or fresh fruit juices are the healthiest option; squeeze your own. Avoid fruit juice concentrates as they are high in sugar. Tea and coffee should be taken without sugar and use semi-skimmed or skimmed milk. Tea, coffee and some fizzy drinks contain caffeine which should be minimised if possible. Try and cut down on the number of cups you have a day or switch to caffeine free fizzy drinks or de-caffeinated brands which at least contain caffeine in much smaller quantities. You will avoid the peaks and troughs of energy that you get as a result of high caffeine intake
- Alcohol has a high sugar content, so this should be taken into account when looking at how much sugar you have on a daily basis. Stick to low sugar alcoholic drinks. For example, drink dry rather than sweet wines or ciders and minimise liqueurs and sweet mixers. Most soft drinks are available in diet form, which are much lower in calories

Myth:	Eating fat is always bad for you
Myth buster:	There are "good" fats and called monounsaturated fats and omega 3, which help protect you against heart attack and stroke. You should include these in your diet

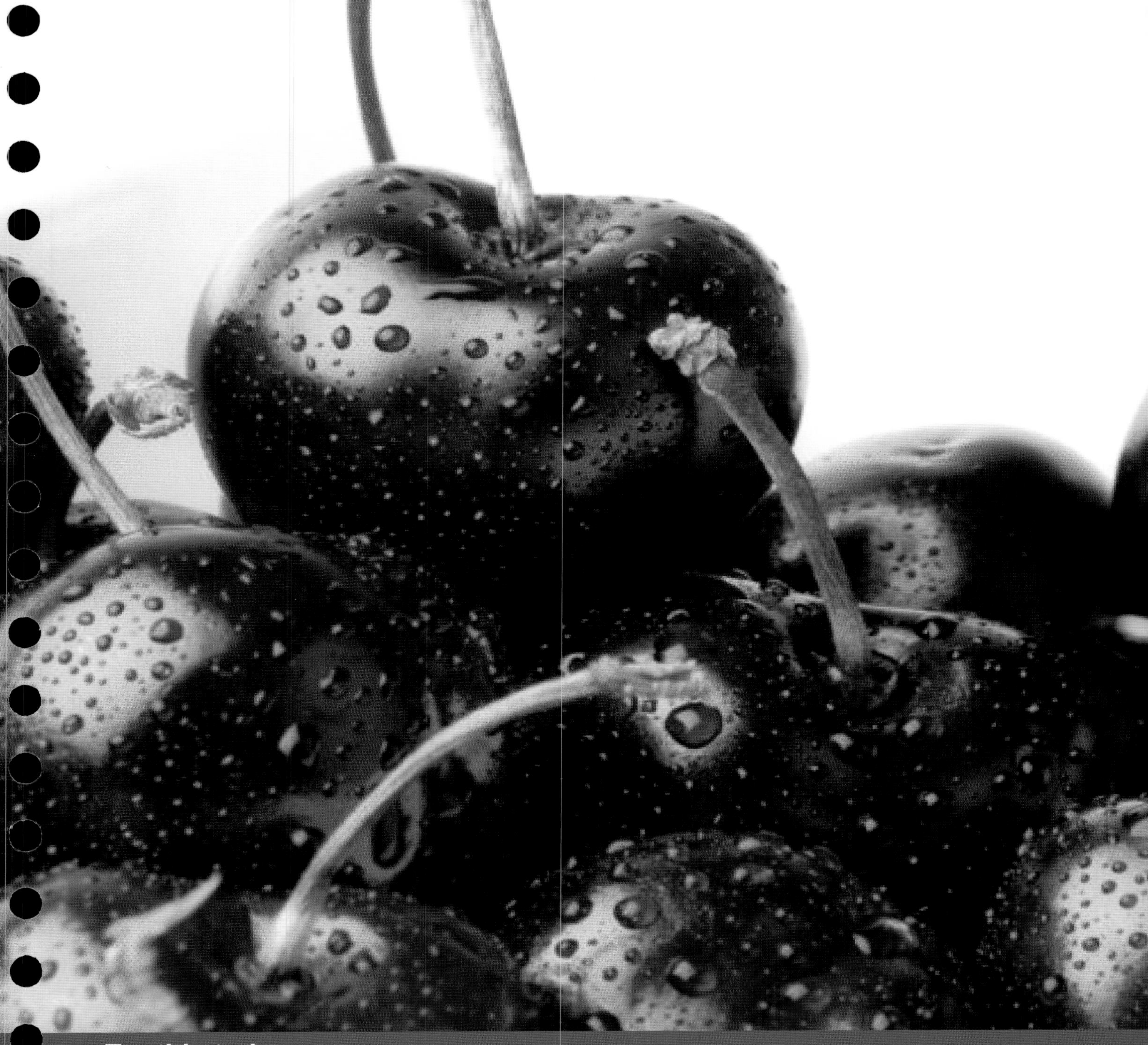

Try this today

Pick one of the following and make a start today:

- Eat healthy snacks
- Cook a meal from fresh ingredients
- Eat 3 pieces of fruit
- Make a salad without using lettuce or cucumber (if you are low on ideas try a simple salsa by dicing a red pepper and an orange and serve with no dressing. Alternatively sliced pears, watercress and pecans go really well together)
- Eat a portion of fish
- Drink 6 cups of fluid other than tea or coffee
- Eat meals of the recommended portion size
- Cook without adding salt
- Sit at a different place at the table
- Wear a funny hat while you are eating (no, just kidding)

Don't cut out carbohydrates

Ironically when most people go on diets, the thing that they try to cut out is the carbohydrate. It is not the carbohydrate that you should focus on but what you put on it, in the form of butter, cheese or rich sauces and dressings.

Carbohydrates exist in 2 forms: simple carbohydrates such as sugars and complex or "good" carbohydrates such as bread, cereals, potatoes, rice and pasta.

Sugars are bad for you; they are high in calories and have no nutritional value but, complex carbohydrate if eaten in slow release form such as brown bread, potatoes, oats, brown rice or pasta, are really good at satisfying hunger and they fill you up for longer than any other food group.

Your appetite centre in the brain requires twice as much fat to switch off the hunger signals as it does carbohydrate. Not only will the fat fill you up for a shorter amount of time, but it will give you many more calories.

You can eat it all

A healthy diet does not restrict you from eating from any of the food groups. In fact it positively encourages you to eat from ALL of them. Life is too short not to have any pleasures!

Eating healthily does however require you to eat *fewer* of the things that are bad for you as they are high in calories and contain no nutritional value. Eat chocolate, eat cakes, eat sweets and biscuits but save these things for occasional treats. Focus on eating those things that are good for you as the mainstay of your diet.

Replacing the high calorie foods with lower calorie options means that rather than eating less to be healthy or to lose weight, you can still eat plenty.

Make sure that you eat as varied a diet as possible, choosing widely from all of the different food groups. This way not only is your diet interesting but full of a broader range of vitamins and minerals.

Look at your portion sizes

Sensible eating does not encourage you to count calories. It does not require you to weigh your food. It does however ask you to look at portion size, as a good balance of far too much food will still leave you overweight.

Prepare your own food

You should prepare food yourself as much as you can, in order to avoid the high fat/salt content of pre-packaged or ready made meals.

Eat together as a family

Your children learn their healthy eating habits from you. If they see you eating well, they will follow. This will imprint healthy ideals on them for life. Meal time is also a good family bonding time.

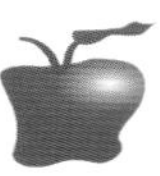

How and when to eat

There are no rules about when is the best time to eat. Food eaten at night is not more likely to be converted into fat. However research does show that those who skip meals in the day and eat late at night tend to be more overweight than those who eat regularly through the day.

More important than when you eat is your total intake of food over the day.

Always eat three meals a day

Missing a meal is the temptation if you are keen to lose weight. This will lead to cravings for sugary things. These are not only high in calories but have lower nutritional value.

Eating a sweet snack when craving sugar will cause a sudden rise in your blood sugar, followed by a rebound fall. You will be temporarily sated only to find yourself craving yet more sugar.

If you eat regular meals, you shouldn't get so many cravings and so it's much easier to avoid falling into the binge and snack trap.

Eat plenty of slow release carbohydrates

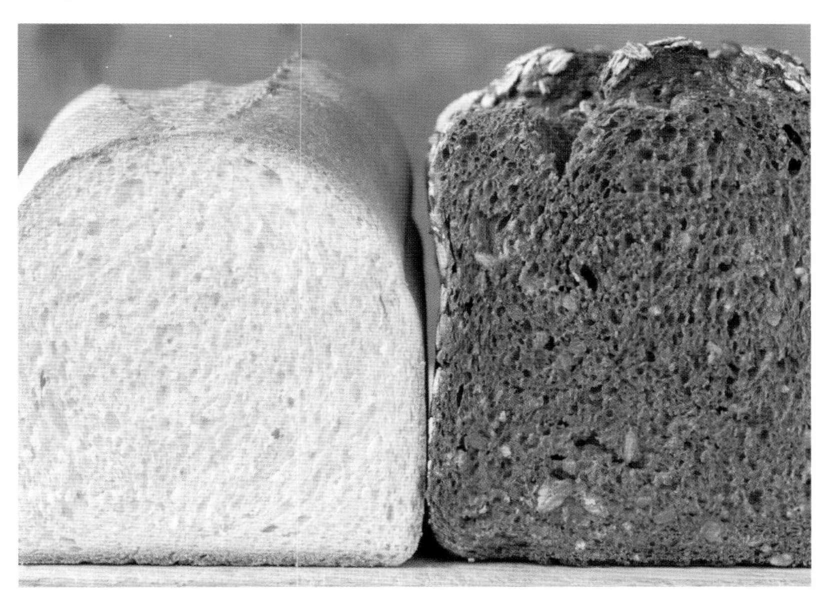

If you eat slow release carbohydrates such as oaty cereals for your breakfast, (take a look at my web site for my oaty breakfast cereal recipe on www.healthcompass.co.uk. My daughter calls it my "horse food" and has glued a picture of a horse to the top of the box. I prefer to call it my "race horse food." Did you ever see a race horse that didn't have a beautiful coat and well toned legs? It could be you...), jacket potatoes, brown rice or brown bread as a regular part of your diet, they will release their energy in a controlled way over a period of hours and you tend not to get the sugar swings, which cause cravings and the need to snack.

This way of eating is also good if you are someone who has peaks and troughs of energy during the day and can be very helpful for some women around the time of their period (try this in combination with less caffeine and alcohol).

What about snacks?

If you are someone who needs to eat between meals, then try using a cereal bar, a handful of unsalted nuts and raisins, chopped raw vegetables, a yoghurt or a piece of fruit such as a banana as an alternative to crisps or sweets. It'll satisfy you for longer and has far better nutritional value. Carry your healthy snacks around with you so that you have access to them when you need them. If you are hungry and need a quick fix, if you don't have them, you will be tempted to buy something unhealthy.

A guide to portions

Have you noticed how many super-size packs and king-size bars there are on the shop shelves? When we eat out, many eateries serve enormous plates of food. Large has become the norm. For many people this has meant they have lost their bench mark of what a normal sized portion is.

Your body gets used to whatever sized meal it is presented with on a regular basis. This means that if you routinely eat a large amount, you will need more to fill you up. The good news however is that the same works in reverse. If you reset your body to eat smaller quantities, you will eventually be satisfied by this amount.

If you suddenly make big changes to the quantity of food you have on your plate, you will of course feel hungry. This is one of the reasons why crash dieting is so difficult to maintain. If however you gradually introduce changes to your portion size, then your body will adjust accordingly and the change in your appetite will be much less noticeable.

A portion guide will give you some idea of how much of each of the foods you should be eating and in what quantities. Use as wide a selection of different foods from the various groups as you can, in order to maintain balance to your diet. You can use the guide on the following pages to help you fill in your Diet Diary in the Personal Health Plan at the back of the book on page 133.

What are your recommended daily allowances?

5 portions of fruit and vegetables

2-3 portions of milk and dairy foods (low fat varieties if possible)

2-3 portions proteins such as meat/fish/nuts/eggs/pulses

7-8 portions of carbohydrates such as bread/cereals/potatoes/rice/pasta

2 portions fatty/sugary foods such as butter/oily dressings/sweets

Obviously there will need to be some flexibility in this. If you were going out for a meal or breaking your routine in some way, then it is almost inevitable that you will exceed your daily amount on that particular day. You can compensate for this by saving up your allowances for the unhealthy things either before or after the event. It's a good idea if you are unfamiliar with this concept to try and be strict with this in the beginning, but as you get used to the idea of what a proper portion size is, you can be a bit more flexible.

How much is a portion?

Fruit and vegetables (5 portions a day)

Whole fresh fruit such as apples, pears, oranges, peaches and bananas……...	1 whole fruit
Fruit juice……………………..	1 small glass
Small fruit…………………….	7 strawberries, 12 grapes, 2 plums, 2 kiwi fruit
Stewed fruit………………….	4 large tablespoons
Dried fruit such as raisins………………………..	1 baby box
Green salad…………………..	1 small bowl
Vegetables such as peas, broccoli, carrots, cabbage, beans and peppers………..	2 large tablespoons

"My doctor told me to stop having intimate dinners for 4; unless there are 3 other people"

Orson Welles

Milk and dairy foods (2-3 portions a day)

Milk, skimmed or semi-skimmed...........	1 medium glass
Yoghurt, low fat................................	1 small pot
Cheese, low fat (Brie, Edam, Camembert, Smoked Austrian, and reduced fat Cheddar)..........................	1 matchbox size
Cream cheese, light...........................	2 small match boxes
Cottage cheese.................................	1 large pot (200g)
Fromage frais, light............................	1 small pot

Protein (2-3 portions a day)

Lean cut beef, pork, ham, chicken, fish...	3 slices, each about the size of a pack of playing cards
Eggs...	2
Baked beans....................................	5 tablespoons
Nuts or peanut butter.........................	2 tablespoons
Lentils..	4 tablespoons cooked

Myth:	Foods marked "low fat" help you lose weight
Myth buster:	Not always. If the food you choose is marked low fat but is high in sugar, the item may still be packed with calories. Make sure you read the label looking at both fat and sugar.

Carbohydrate (7-8 portions a day)

Crumpet, muffin, muesli bar................	1
Bagel..	½
Bread roll.......................................	½ large
Bread/toast.....................................	1 large slice
Pitta bread......................................	1 mini
Crackers...	3
Crisp bread.....................................	4
Plain naan bread.............................	1 small
Weetabix...	1
Muesli..	2 tablespoons
Breakfast cereal such as Cornflakes, Rice Crispies, Branflakes..................	3 tablespoons
Rice (plain boiled)...........................	2 heaped tablespoons
Pasta (plain boiled)..........................	3 heaped tablespoons
Potatoes...	2 egg sized

Sugary foods (a maximum of 1 portion a day or 7 a week)

Sugar..	3 teaspoons
Jam/honey.......................................	1 heaped teaspoon
Ice cream...	1 small scoop
Plain biscuit......................................	2
Slice of cake/doughnut/Danish..............	½
Chocolate bars..................................	1 small/2 mini
Sweets...	1 small tube/bag

Fatty foods (a maximum of 2 portions a day)

Butter, margarine, cooking oil................	1 teaspoon
Low fat spread..................................	2 teaspoons
Mayonnaise.......................................	1 teaspoon
Low calorie mayonnaise.......................	2 teaspoons
Salad cream......................................	1 tablespoon
Gravy/white sauce.............................	1 tablespoon
Crisps (low fat)..................................	1 small packet
Savoury pastry..................................	½
Cream...	1 tablespoon

Rich fatty foods are like destiny. They too shape our ends"

Author unknown

A word on salt

Too much salt in your diet can lead to high blood pressure. The recommended daily allowance is 6g salt or 2.5g sodium a day. Most adults eat 9g or more of salt a day. Pre-packaged and ready made meals are particularly high in salt. It is worth being really careful about salt in particular if you have a personal or family history of high blood pressure, stroke, heart disease or diabetes.

Here are some things you can do to help keep the salt low in your diet:

- Avoid junk foods
- Prepare you own meals as much as possible from fresh ingredients. If you do buy ready meals or canned vegetables make sure you choose the varieties low in salt
- Cook without adding salt to food
- Make your dining table a salt free zone
- Use low salt stock cubes
- Check the labels on food packaging before buying

Your guide to food labelling

In order understand what food labels mean you need to know what the recommended daily allowance of each of the ingredients is for you. Here is a guide:

Table to show recommended daily allowances in men and women in the UK

Nutrient	Men	Women
Calories	2,500	2,000
Fat	95g	70g
Salt	6g (2.5g sodium)	5g (2g sodium)
Sugar	70g	50g

It is a legal requirement that all packaged foods are labelled. You should therefore be able to work out exactly what is in your chosen food from the label. Larger quantities of foods are labelled per serving and smaller quantities per 100g. If you compare this to your recommended daily allowance, you can calculate what proportion that food contains.

For example:

Large quantity	Small quantity
30g fat	3g fat
1.5g salt (0.625g sodium)	0.25g salt (0.1g sodium)
10g sugar	1g sugar

Food labelling should also contain details of colourings and preservatives.

Avoid foods whose labels say “artificial colouring added” or details in its list of ingredients several colours followed by a number, for example Quinoline yellow (E104). Choose foods that use natural colourings such as chlorella, carotene and annatto.

Artificial preservatives include monosodium glutamate, monopotassium glutamate, nitrates, alum, sodium osinate, benzoic acid and benzoates. Choose more foods that are additive and preservative free or that use Citric acid and Ascorbic acid as preservatives as they are natural anti-oxidants and harmless.

The Cholesterol story

Cholesterol is the David and Victoria Beckham of the health press. Everyone seems to be talking about it. It is a fatty substance; one of a group of blood fats or "lipids." Our bodies make it in the liver or get it directly from "saturated" fats, such as found in butter, cream, lard, suet, dripping, ghee, fatty meat, eggs, coconut and palm oil, kidneys, liver and certain shellfish such as prawns.

The most common cause for having a cholesterol level that is too high is from eating too much saturated fat, but can also be due to thyroid or kidney problems or can be inherited.

Doctors worry if you have a high cholesterol level as too much can clog your arteries and can increase your risk of heart disease or stroke. Your risk of suffering from one of these conditions is multiplied if you also have other risk factors such as smoking, diabetes or high blood pressure, or if you are overweight, lead a sedentary lifestyle, are from South Asia or have a history of heart attack or stroke in a family member.

What are the other types of blood fat?

The blood lipids incorporate several types including cholesterol and a type of fat called a triglyceride. Triglycerides are found in dairy products, cooking oils and meat and are found in higher concentrations in the blood of people who are overweight, drink a lot of alcohol or eat a lot of fatty or sugary foods. Those with high triglyceride levels have a higher risk of heart disease and stroke.

Have you heard of LDL and HDL cholesterol?

Cholesterol is transported around the body using special carriers called lipoproteins. High density lipoproteins (HDL) are used to carry excess cholesterol to the liver. We call HDL "good" cholesterol as it removes cholesterol from the blood stream where it can damage the arteries.

Low density lipoproteins (LDL) are used to carry cholesterol from the liver, to the arteries, where excess can be deposited. It is a "bad" cholesterol, as deposits of cholesterol can accumulate to block the arteries. Obstruction of blood flow to the heart as a result of cholesterol build up can result in heart attack and angina and the same process in the arteries of the brain can lead to stroke.

How do we measure cholesterol?

Doctors use a blood test to measure your cholesterol level. Your doctor will be able to tell from this test what the levels of cholesterol, triglycerides, HDL and LDL are in your blood. Some pharmacies also now offer a finger prick blood test. This test is limited in that it only measures total cholesterol level and not any other of the blood fats, but can be useful as a screening tool, before you go and see your doctor. If this test is normal, it is likely that one done by your GP will be too.

The first time you have your blood test your doctor will ask you to have your test "fasting." This means to have your blood taken having had nothing to eat or drink other than water, from midnight the night before your sample is taken. This is because food and drink (with the exception of water) can influence your blood triglyceride levels. As long as you have a normal triglyceride level, subsequent blood tests can be done without fasting.

Ideally you should have low total cholesterol, low LDL and triglyceride level and a high HDL level.

Doctors can use the ratio of your total cholesterol level to HDL level to work out your risk of heart disease or stroke. The higher the ratio is, the higher your risk.

The figure you should aim for if you have already had a heart attack or stroke is:

- a total cholesterol level of below 4
- a total cholesterol to HDL level of below 4

How can my diet influence my cholesterol level?

Eating healthily can reduce your cholesterol levels by approximately 10%. This varies from person to person. The following guide should help. You should:

- Reduce your total fat intake
- Decrease the amount of saturated fats you eat and replace them with monounsaturated fats (such as olive and rapeseed oil, seeds, some margarines, avocado and nuts such as hazelnuts, cashews, pistachios, peanuts, almonds), and polyunsaturated fats (such as corn oil, sunflower oil, soya oil, seeds and some nuts such as pine and walnuts).
- Decrease the trans fats you eat (found in processed fats such as in cakes, biscuits, pastries and crackers or foods that contain hydrogenated oils such as hard margarines)
- Eat oily fish regularly (once a week if you are otherwise healthy or 2 or 3 times a week if you have had a heart attack or stroke) as it is rich in omega 3

How can replacing one fat with another help?

Different fats have different effects on your blood lipids. Some are good for you and so are important to include in your diet. Here is a guide:

- Saturated fats can increase your total cholesterol and your LDL (bad cholesterol) levels. Cut these out of your diet
- Monounsaturated fats can lower your LDL (bad cholesterol) level but do not lower your HDL (good cholesterol) levels so these are the best fats to eat
- Polyunsaturated fats can lower both your LDL (bad cholesterol) and HDL (good cholesterol) levels
- Omega-3 lowers your triglyceride levels and should be incorporated into your diet

What is omega 3?

Omega 3 is a polyunsaturated fat found in oily fish such as herring, mackerel, tuna, pilchards, trout and salmon. It is also found in eggs and certain oils such as flax seed and rape seed oils and in some nuts and seeds such as walnuts and flax seeds.

It helps your body by reducing your blood triglyceride level which if too high can increase your risk of heart attack and stroke. It also helps prevent your blood from clotting and helps regulate the rhythm of your heart.

Are there any other ways I can reduce my blood cholesterol?

- Increase the fibre in your diet by eating plenty of fresh fruit and vegetables. Aim for at least 5 portions a day. Fibre "soaks up" cholesterol
- Replace saturated fats in your diet with sterol or stanol enriched foods such as found in some margarines, soft cheeses and yoghurts. This can be helpful if you are unable to take medication
- Exercise regularly

Will I need to take medication?

Your doctor can use special “predictive tables” which take into account your age, sex, blood pressure and smoking status, to predict your risk of heart disease over the next 10 years.

The higher the risk, the more likely your doctor will want to prescribe medication to help lower your cholesterol level. This might include if you have a strong history of heart disease or stroke in other family members at a young age.

Incorporating exercise and some of the healthy eating ideas from the previous page into your life could lower your cholesterol level enough to prevent you from having to take medication. In addition, if you reduce other risk factors you might have for heart disease or stroke such as stopping smoking, losing weight and controlling your blood pressure, there may be no need for you to take medication. Your doctor may want to give you a 3 month trial of “lifestyle changes” before prescribing.

Even if your doctor does recommend medication, it is still important to eat healthily and exercise regularly.

Other medical conditions can increase your risk of heart attack and stroke. If you suffer from one of these, your doctor will recommend that you take medication to lower your risk even if you have a normal cholesterol level. Examples of these are diabetes and peripheral arterial disease. If you have already had a heart attack or stroke, it is also advisable to take medication as this lowers your risk of having a further event.

Conversely if you have a high cholesterol level but no other risk factors for heart attack or stroke, you may not need to take medication as your overall risk maybe low.

What are the medications my doctor might recommend?

Statins

This is the most common group of drugs used to treat high cholesterol levels. They can reduce your total cholesterol level by up to 20% and your LDL level by up to 30%.

Statins can reduce the risk of heart attack or stroke by about a quarter.
It is now possible to buy low dose statins over the counter at your pharmacist.

Side effects include nausea, muscles aches, diarrhoea and headaches. You should not drink grapefruit juice while taking a statin and you cannot take them while pregnant or breastfeeding or suffering with liver disease.

If you are unable to take statins there are other cholesterol lowering medications available. Examples of these are:

- Fibrates
- Ezetimibe
- Drugs that bind bile acids
- Nicotinic acid drugs

What else can I do to improve my diet?

Learn to cook

I like this one, because it's such an easy thing to do and the health benefits can be huge.

Many families now have two parents who work. With less time in the day, the temptation is to reach for a ready made meal. The disadvantage of this is not only are many high in salt and fat but we are becoming de-skilled at cooking. As a result of this many of our younger generation, who would have learnt their cooking skills from their parents are unable to do so and grow up not knowing even the basics of cooking.

In reality, I find that when I use a ready made meal, it takes almost as long to get sorted out as throwing together a quick bowl of pasta and a salad.

If you have the skills, make sure you use them. The more fresh ingredients you use the better. You don't need to be a domestic God or Goddess. Often the simplest meals are the healthiest. Make a resolution to cut down or stop using ready made meals. If you do need to use them occasionally, make sure you read the food label and buy those that are low in fat and salt.

Teach your children how to cook if you know how. This will be an invaluable life skill.

If you don't know how to cook, there are some great adult and children's cookery courses available, which you can find on the internet. There are also some wonderful learn to cook books on the market. Have a look at the BBC's children's learn to cook book by Joanna Farrow: "Ready Steady Cook."

> Beth's top tip:
> Girls love a man who can cook. If you want to improve your popularity with the ladies; get into the kitchen.

Keep a Diet Diary

A helpful exercise when embarking on a healthy lifestyle plan is to keep a Diet Diary for a week. Make a note of everything you eat and drink over that period of time, including snacks and drinks.

It's really important to be honest with yourself for this one. In this way, you can identify where your weak points are and replace them with healthier alternatives. Have a look at the Diet Diary in your Personal Health Plan, on page 133, which you shows you how easy it is to do.

There are more calories in an alco-pop than there are in a kit-kat

Mark's story

Mark is 50 years old and a long distance lorry driver. He has just been told by his GP that he has a slightly raised cholesterol level. In addition to this a recent blood pressure check has shown that his blood pressure is borderline high. One of the things that his GP has told him may make a difference is improving his diet.

Mark has driven lorries for 25 years and has roughly followed the same routine. He keeps a Diet Diary for a week, which gives us plenty to work on!

Mark starts work early each morning at around 6 o'clock and doesn't feel like breakfast at that time. He gets on the road and makes a service station pit stop for a fry up, every week day. He usually has several items through the day on which he snacks, including chocolate bars (king-size) and crisps. He stops at a wayside café or service station for a burger or sandwich for lunch and then eats a meat and 2 veg. supper when he gets home. On the road he drinks strong coffee with 2 sugars, and at home has 2 or 3 cans of lager every evening, in addition to which he drinks 2 or 3 pints of lager on a couple of nights, when out with his friends. He doesn't smoke. His only exercise is loading and unloading his truck, which can be strenuous at times. He is 13kg (2 stone) overweight.

Mark is concerned to hear that having a raised cholesterol level, in addition to high blood pressure puts him at risk of stroke and heart disease. He has a friend who recently had a heart attack when he was in his early 50s and so is keen to make some changes.

He acknowledges that he is overweight, but he has a large appetite and is not keen to tackle this at this point. Neither does he want to exercise. He agrees that changing what he eats to be more "heart friendly" would be a good start.

Mark makes some changes to his diet. He swaps his fry up for a healthier breakfast. He starts making his own muesli style cereal, in which he includes walnuts, which are a rich source of omega 3, (which is good for your heart) and dried fruit, (which is a good source of fibre and so is good at lowering cholesterol levels, as are oats). He prepares this in a plastic tub at the beginning of the week and takes a smaller pot of it with him in his cab. He can then eat it when he is ready for it. He swaps from full fat to semi-skimmed milk on his cereal and in his coffee and he manages to cut out one of the sugars. His wife makes him a sandwich, which she prepares the night before, so that he can take it for his lunch, when he leaves early in the morning. This means he avoids the high fat burgers that he normally has for lunch, which are also high in salt and can elevate blood pressure. His wife buys benecol margarine, which he uses on his bread instead of butter. One day a week he has tuna in his sandwich, as oily fish is a great source of omega 3. He is not a great fan of oily fish, so supplements his diet with a daily omega 3 capsule. At night his wife prepares red meat only twice a week and on the other nights she cooks chicken and occasionally white fish. She grills, rather than fries when she cooks and avoids chips, cooking more boiled and jacket potatoes. Mark exchanges one of his nightly lagers for a glass of red wine. He takes his healthy snacks with him when he goes to work, so he isn't tempted by the service station bars. When he does buy a chocolate bar (he still has one every day!) he buys a regular size.

After 3 months Mark's cholesterol level is slightly improved and so is his blood pressure, and much to his amazement and delight he has lost 3kg (half a stone) in weight.

My thoughts

Prevention is better than cure. What we are doing with Mark is getting in to help, before any damage is done. The combination of his sedentary lifestyle, with high fat diet, high blood pressure and raised cholesterol mean he is at greatly increased risk of developing heart problems or stroke. The fact that his blood pressure is raised at such an early age would suggest that his lifestyle is already taking its toll.

Motivation always helps. Mark is well motivated in some areas and not in others. We have to work with this. There is no point at this stage focusing on him exercising or losing weight, if he doesn't have the inclination. We will make the changes when he is ready.

What is interesting is that many of the changes that we would recommend for him to make in order to get his cholesterol level down are the same as those needed to lower blood pressure. Improving one area will have a knock on effect in others and therefore will multiply your protection. We see this when Mark loses weight without necessarily having worked on this area.

What else can Mark do to improve his cholesterol level when the time is right?

- Exercise, at the recommended level of 30 minutes 5 times a week (unloading his cab could count towards this)
- Lose more weight
- Increase the fibre in his diet by eating more fruit and vegetables
- Eat oily fish once or twice a week (herring, mackerel, pilchards, sardines, salmon, tuna, trout) as they are rich in omega 3 which is good for your heart
- Eat more Soya products
- Swap saturated fats (such as butter, cheese, meat, lard, cream, suet and ghee) and trans fats (such as found in pastries, cakes, biscuits, crackers or hard margarines) for unsaturated fats (such as olive oil, sunflower oil, avocado, nuts, seeds and margarine)

Other things that Mark might consider to make his life more "heart friendly" include:

- Keeping his food salt free (the bacon in his fry ups is a big culprit)
- Decreasing his alcohol level to 3-4 units a night (red wine offers greatest protection to your heart). Note Mark is 50 years old and so alcohol does offer his heart some protection. This protective effect only starts from age 44 years. Keeping one or two days alcohol free would also help

Diet
(From broad bean to runner bean)

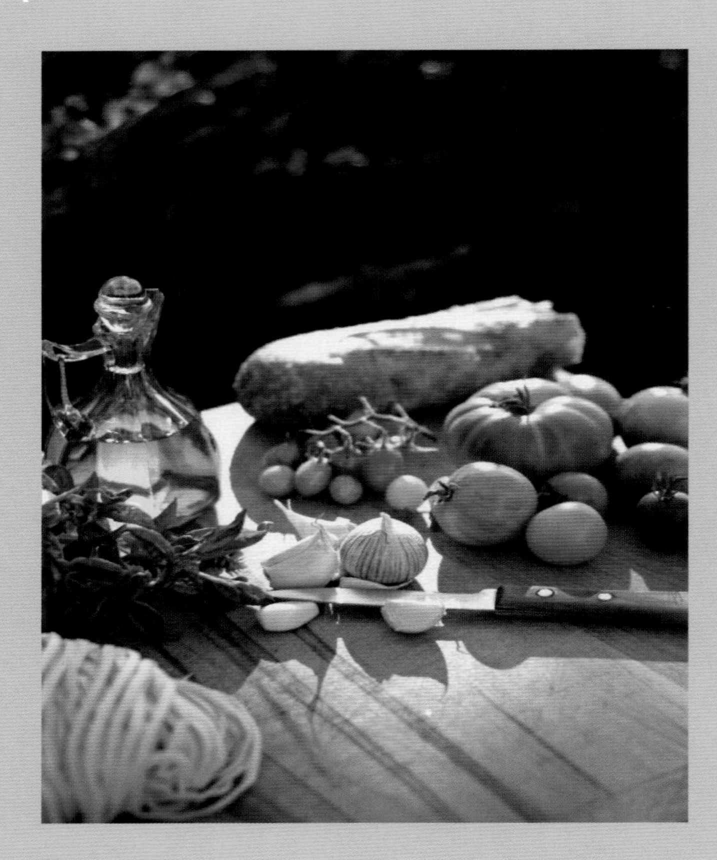

Remember

- Avoid fad diets; think "lifestyle change"
- Eat a balanced diet using all the food groups
- Eat less fatty and sugary foods
- Drink plenty
- Eat your biggest meal in the morning
- Eat regular meals
- Don't snack, but plan your snacks if you can't avoid it
- Watch your portion sizes
- Prepare your meals with fresh ingredients
- Make your table a salt free zone

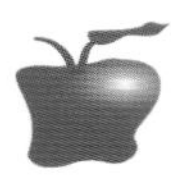

Exercise
(One small step for man; one giant leap for mankind)

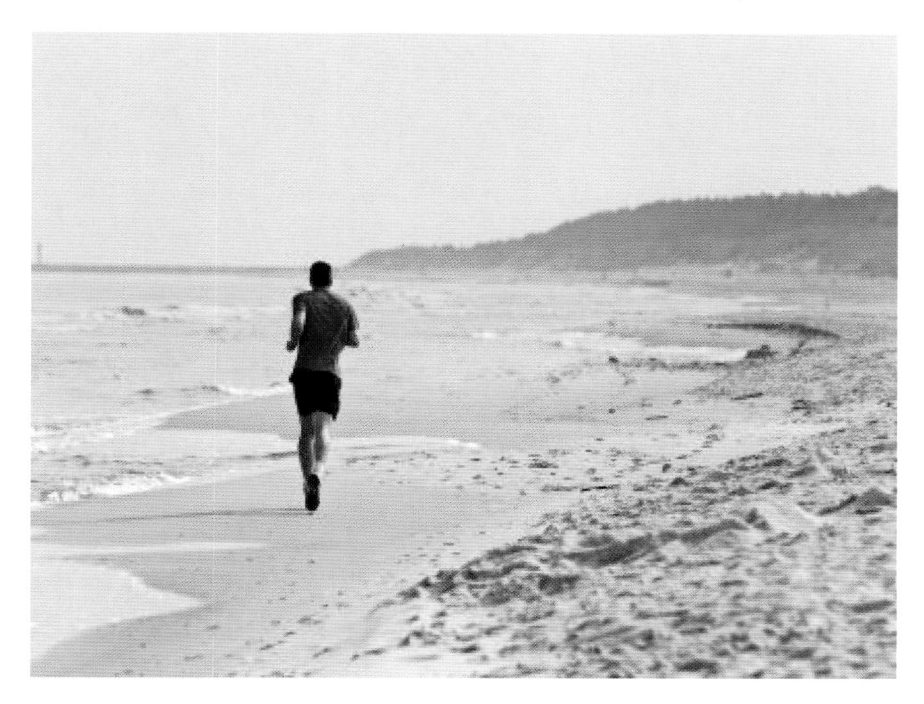

One of my favourite things in life is getting out and exercising. It doesn't matter how; walking, cycling, running, swimming, Tae Kwon-do, gardening, body boarding or kayaking. After years of chipping away, my husband finally persuaded me that a dance class would be fun and we have started to learn to jive. Apart from the fact that I have two left feet and the co-ordination, elegance and finesse of a grizzly bear, I have at least laughed a lot and I really do believe that no matter who and what age you are, it is possible to teach an old dog new tricks.

Don't take life too seriously; get out and exercise and have some fun.

In 1907 the average worker walked for 2 hours before starting work. Many of us drive everywhere these days and most of us spend several hours a day, watching TV or sitting in front of a computer screen rather than spending our time in a more active fashion. Families often have both partners working and tiredness and long hours are a disincentive to get out and exercise.

We are less willing to let our children walk or cycle to school because of the volume of traffic and the perceived risk of "stranger danger." For the same reasons, our children don't go outside all day and play.

The net effect is that as a nation, we have become less active.

Exercise releases the body's own morphine like substances, called "endorphins," which give you a natural high

If you are someone who suffers with low mood or stress, adding regular exercise into your weekly regime, may be all you need to do

"The trouble with jogging is that the ice falls out of your glass"

Martin Hull

Why should I exercise?

In short, because it will make you feel great.

Exercise can prevent or improve many medical conditions. Regular exercise will reduce your risk of heart disease, diabetes and stroke. Even if you have already developed one of these conditions, exercise can reduce your risk of further problems. It will reduce lung problems including asthma and smokers lung and will improve snoring. It will help back pain and arthritis; your joints will feel freer and less painful.

Mood swings or depression could be a thing of the past. Exercise is a great way to improve self confidence. You will feel fitter, stronger and more healthy. Your energy levels and quality of sleep will improve.

Friendships made through exercise tend to be strong. Exercising with colleagues or family can improve these relationships and develops powerful and lasting bonds.

In combination with a well balanced diet, regular exercise can help you lose weight. It tones your body, making your physique firmer and reducing cellulite. It stimulates blood and lymph circulation, reducing the risk of varicose veins and leg ulcers and giving your skin a healthy glow.

Make a start today. It doesn't have to be much. Do one small thing. Get off the bus a stop early and walk the extra 10 minutes to work. Walk to the shop to get your morning paper instead of driving. Take the stairs instead of the lift. Use this as your starting point. Build gradually. You are capable of great things.

How much exercise do I need to do?

The recommended level of exercise for adults is 30 minutes of exercise, 5 times a week. For children it is an hour every day. If you are exercising to lose weight then you should aim to do an hour a day. Ideally exercising should be like brushing your teeth. You wouldn't think about going to bed without having done it.

Exercise should be performed at a level to get your heart rate up in a sustained way for the full 30 minutes (unless you are taking medication which slows down your heart rate such as beta blockers). You should feel warm and slightly out of breath but not so breathless that you have difficulty speaking (this is called the talk test).

Any exercise is better than no exercise. So although 30 minutes five times a week is your ideal, if you can do only half of this or less, it is still better than nothing at all. There is good evidence to show that less than this is still beneficial. So do what you can. You may be able to increase what you are doing at a later date.

You may need to build up to the recommended level if you currently do no exercise. You may have to split your sessions, for instance 30 minutes once daily, could be 15 minutes twice a day for 5 days. It may be easier to fit your exercise in around a busy lifestyle or around the limitations of an illness in this way. Dividing your sessions like this is as beneficial to you as doing your whole exercise session in one sitting. Pushing your exercise sessions together is better than doing nothing. So if for example you work long hours during the week, doing 2 lots of longer sessions at the weekend, would work well.

What kind of exercise should I do?

The most important message to get across when deciding what exercise you should do, is that if you are to maintain it for life it needs to be enjoyable or fun.

Depending on what kind of exercise you take, will depend on whether this will be sufficient on its own to help you lose weight. Exercise may just be a way for you to improve your cardiovascular fitness and feeling of wellbeing.

If you suffer with a pre-existing medical problem or if you are extremely overweight, your condition will probably benefit from exercise, but you should check with your doctor before you start exercising and build up gradually.

"Aerobic" exercise such as running, swimming, cycling, dance and aerobics is good for weight loss. This needs to be done at a level that you feel warm and slightly out of breath, for at least an hour a day in order that you lose weight.

Gym based exercise is better for muscle toning and tends not to lose you weight, however this is still beneficial for your cardiovascular system.

Weight bearing exercise such as running or brisk walking is good for you if you suffer from, or have a family history of osteoporosis.

Non weight-bearing exercise such as swimming, cycling or aqua-aerobics is better for you if you suffer with joint problems or are overweight.

Exercise such as Pilates, yoga or Tai chi are also good if you are overweight, have joint problems, are pregnant or need stress relief. There is a misconception that these forms of exercise are gentle. Certainly they don't get your pulse rate up as running or swimming might and they won't on their own help you lose weight. However they can be incredibly challenging and the benefits can be enormous, encouraging good posture, relief of back and neck pain, improved muscle strength, sleep and digestion. By and large you can do them to your own level and they can be done at any age.

There are many activities that we do as part of our daily lives that could count towards our exercise sessions. Walking to work, climbing stairs, gardening, vacuuming, can all be taken into account as long as they are done energetically enough to get your heart rate up in a sustained fashion.

It may be that all you have to do to achieve your target level of recommended exercise is to increase the vigour with which you do certain of your normal daily activities or to tailor an activity that you already do. For instance, taking the stairs instead of the lift; walking to get the morning milk and paper instead of taking the car; walking the children to school, instead of driving them.

Have a look at: www.cyclescheme.co.uk a government scheme set up to encourage employees to cycle to work. This scheme allows you to save up to 50% on the cost of a new bicycle or motorised cycle.

"If your dog is fat, you're not getting enough exercise"

Author unknown

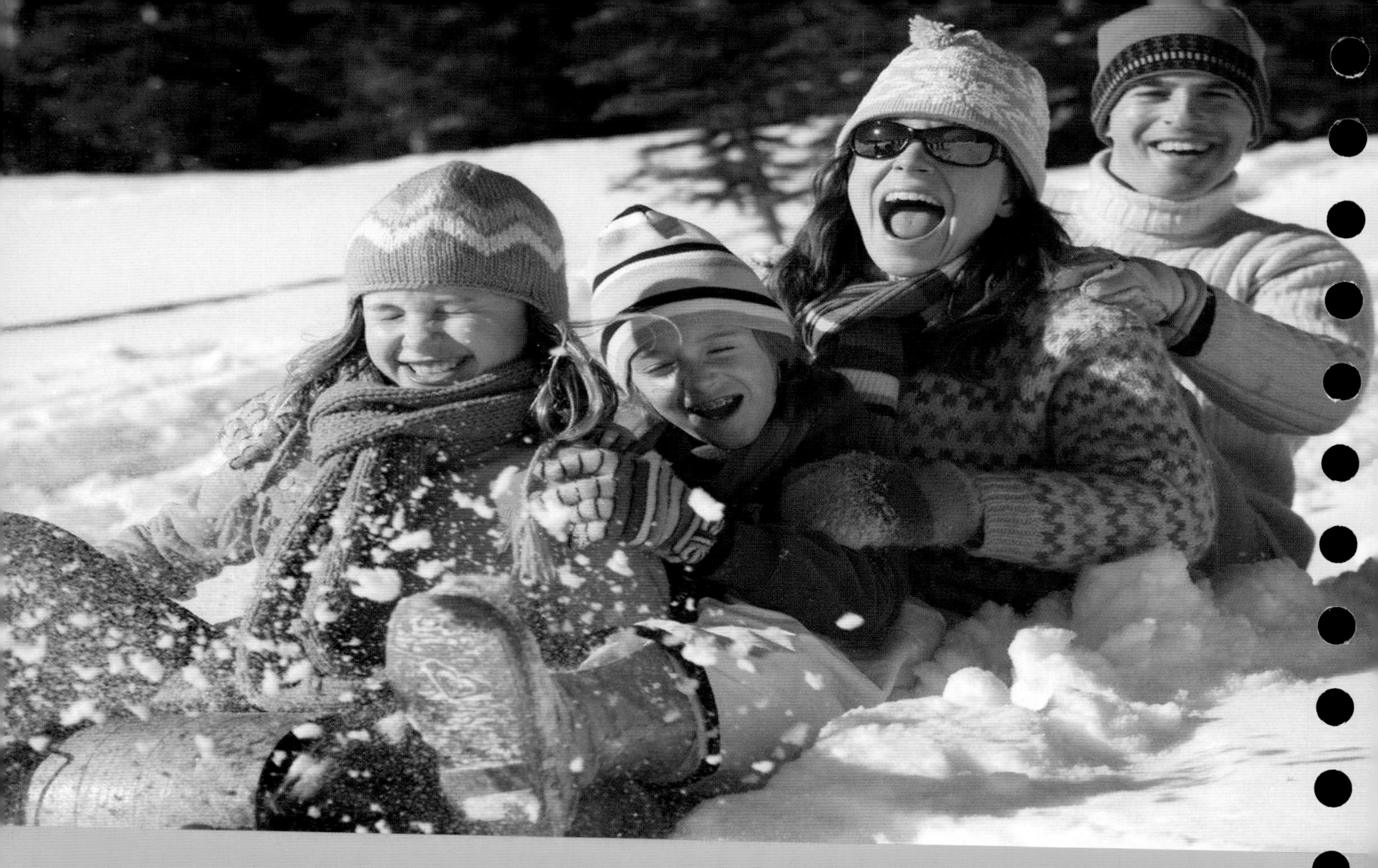

Exercise with your family

You may want to choose an exercise that you can do together as a family.

If you are a city dweller and don't have access to the countryside or the sea, most areas now have swimming pools or ice rinks that are a great way to get the family involved in exercise.

Most people living in built up areas have access to a local park. If you have a dog with you, not only is it a great excuse to get out in all weathers, but the kids love running around after a dog. Take a picnic or a cricket bat along. Rounders is easy to play, and the children love it. Think about getting together with neighbours and starting a family soft ball or football league. My local Tae Kwon-do group runs family classes and my whole family train together in the same class.

Check out your local tennis or running club, which will usually welcome children. Orienteering clubs run courses of different levels from toddlers to serious competitors when they organise most events and running events usually have children's fun-runs attached and make a really nice day out. A trampoline in the garden or basket ball hoop on a wall is a good way for your children to exercise if you have limited space.

If you live near the sea, think about body boarding, surfing, kayaking or sailing. Spending time with your children or partner doing fun activities is enormously bonding and it also sets your children's blueprint for exercising for the rest of their lives. If you are doing fun, sporty activities with your teenagers, it can keep them close both physically and emotionally.

 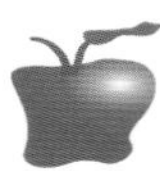

Geo-caching is a really fun way to introduce your children to walking and map reading and involves following clues, using a GPS (Global Positioning System), to boxes containing gifts, hidden about the countryside. Take a look at the web site on: www.geocache.co.uk

If you live in the Southwest with access to Dartmoor, a more local version of this is letterboxing, involving using a compass, to locate boxes containing stamps which are hidden at various locations about Dartmoor. For information as to how to get involved, look at : www.letterboxingondartmoor.co.uk

If you don't know how to read a compass or map, your local Youth Hostel will probably run courses at reasonable cost.

Have you thought about climbing? There are climbing centres available in both cities and rural areas with sometimes both indoor and outdoor climbing walls. Often affiliated climbing clubs will organise trips to rural venues. This can be a great way for the whole family to have fun and can be a really good way of getting to see different parts of the country.

What about learning a martial art? This is a great way to learn an invaluable life skill, whilst improving your self confidence, strength, balance, co-ordination, flexibility and cardiovascular fitness. Some disciplines such as Tae Kwon-do run family classes.

Beth's top tip:
Children love walking as long as you make it fun. Make the walk exciting; call it a mission or an adventure. Give them things to look for: this can be anything, for example red cars or wild life, or you can even hide treats along the way.

Children burn their calories in a different way to adults. Adults take about 2 hours of continuous aerobic exercise such as running, cycling, or swimming, before their fat stores are tapped. However, as soon as children start exercising, they begin to burn off fat. Exercising is therefore a really good way for overweight children to lose weight

"A bear however hard he tries, grows tubby without exercise"

A.A. Milne

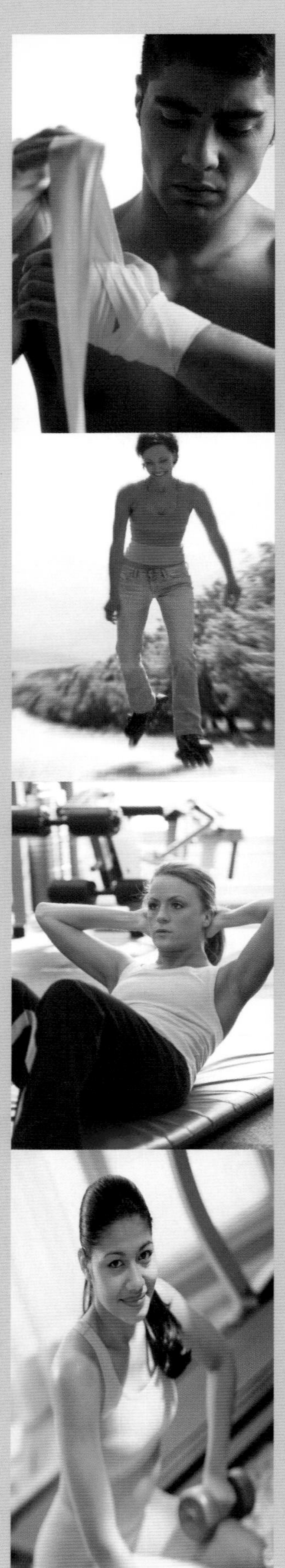

Choose something you will enjoy

Look at the Sport England web site that lists an A-Z of sports, to see if you can find something that interests you on:www.sportengland.org/index/get_active/find_the_sport_for_you.htm

You can mix and match different types of exercise at different times of the week or year to accommodate the seasons. This is called "cross-training." It is not unusual for one type of exercise to benefit another. You will also find that different exercises use different muscle groups and so work a bigger range of muscles. When one set of muscles are tired, this will give you the opportunity to rest that group while continuing to exercise another. This will also give you more options if you are injured. For instance, if your knees are hurting following a long walk or run, you could substitute a swim or cycle.

There are some great national exercise schemes in place:

- If you are interested in walking in a group, contact www.whi.org.uk for information regarding local groups.
- www.bikeforall.net gives you information regarding local cycle facilities including cycle path networks.
- www.swim4fitness.com offers an internet based swim programme that you can tailor to your level and needs.
- www.womensrunningnetwork.co.uk is a national women's running group. The web site will tell you where your nearest group is and inform you of local events. This is great, safe and supportive way for women to get out running and is a good way of making new friends.
- www.britmilfit.com is an organisation with groups running throughout the country providing "an alternative to the lycra clad, Swiss ball using and water-fountain world of the gym." Run by ex army physical fitness instructors it provides fitness training for all levels of ability in twice daily, hour long classes held outdoors in city parks. Classes are held in the spirit that if you are to maintain fitness for any length of time, it needs to be varied and fun.

If you don't enjoy sports, but like the outdoors, how about getting involved in a local volunteer group, clearing woodland, ponds, cycle-ways or footpaths. These activities are often strenuous and can be a fun way to meet new people and keep fit whilst helping the community and environment. Have a look at: www.sustrans.org.uk or contact the National Trust at: www.nationaltrust.org.uk/volunteering/

How should I go about starting to get active?

Start gently and build up gradually. This may be as little as starting off by walking to the end of the road and back. Don't worry, you will build on this. A good rule of thumb is to try and increase your level by 10-20% a week. You may have to go slower than this. Plunging in with a heavy session the first time you go, may injure you and set you back.

With every session you do, make sure you start gently so that your body is warmed up before you go at full throttle. Sudden bursts of vigorous exercise when you are middle aged and unfit could cause angina. Warming up sensibly will also help prevent injury. Don't exercise on a full stomach or when you have a viral infection or a temperature.

Wear the appropriate clothing for the exercise that you are doing. Make sure that if you are walking, you wear good walking boots or running shoes in addition to good insoles if you can. Running shoes have really good inbuilt shock absorbers and when used in addition to insoles provide you with excellent cushioning. This is especially important if you suffer with problems with your feet, ankles, knees, hips or lower back.

If you are aiming to lose weight, try not to be too hung up on weight loss when you first start exercising. As muscle weighs more than fat, sometimes you can experience an initial small weight gain. The way I like to think of the situation at this point is that your body although slightly heavier, is working better metabolically for you. This is the starting point, and from this foundation as your stamina improves and you build up your regime, if you don't increase what you eat, you should eventually lose weight.

If you have never exercised before ask your GP about Exercise Referral Programmes, which can be really helpful when getting started. I will talk about these later.

If you have exercised in the past, but have lost fitness, or if you are aiming for a specific event such as a marathon, think about hiring a personal trainer. They can be really helpful with motivation, if you are having trouble getting going and will be able to design a regime which is specific for you, including nutritional advice.

Most gyms now offer personal trainers as part of their service, and local council run gyms will often charge very reasonable rates. It's worth checking this out first. If you have no luck, try the Register of Exercise Professionals on: www.exerciseregister.org

This site hosts a national list of personal trainers. There are also trainers listed on this site with special interests such as training those with disabilities.

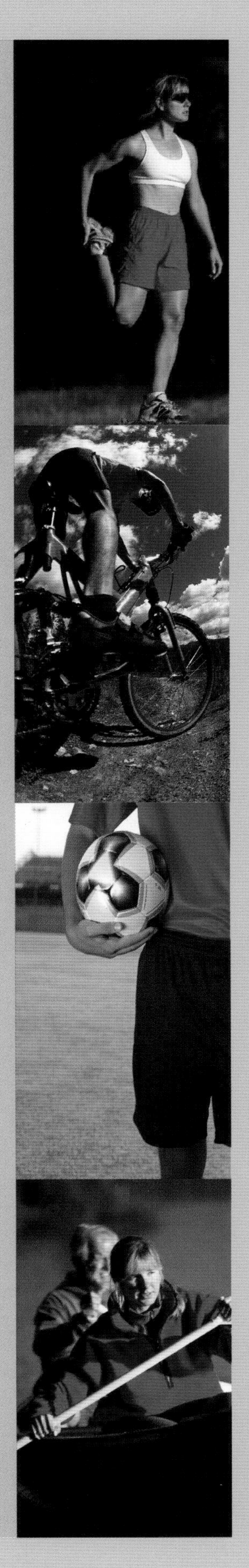

What about exercising when I am pregnant?

Exercise is encouraged if you are pregnant. It can have huge benefits, including reduction of varicose veins, back pain, swelling of your limbs (oedema), and prevention of weight gain, high blood pressure and diabetes.

Exercise during pregnancy can also reduce the length of your labour and decrease complications during labour.

How much and what should I do?

Use a healthy dose of common sense here. As a general rule, any exercise done in moderation, with a few exceptions is OK. If you already do a sport then as long as you avoid exercising to peak physical fitness or to exhaustion, you can continue as you have done previously. You must however expect a decline in your performance as your pregnancy progresses.

If you don't already exercise, then make sure that you build up your exercise levels gradually. Ideal exercises are brisk walking, swimming or aqua-aerobics.

Exercise has been shown to have no adverse effect on the developing baby as long as you take certain precautions. The Royal College of Obstetrician and Gynaecologists have issued the following guidelines:

Basic rules to follow are drink plenty, don't exercise in extreme heat, limit your session to a maximum of 45 minutes and make sure that you have a really good warm up and warm down with each session.

As long as you exercise sensibly, you should encounter no problems. However in the unlikely event that you become excessively breathless, dizzy or have palpitations, have painful uterine contractions, abdominal or pelvic pain, amniotic fluid leak or bleeding or reduced foetal movements, you should stop immediately and consult a doctor.

Sports such as horse riding, cycling, skiing, gymnastics and contact sports should be avoided simply because a fall could damage your baby. Scuba diving and stomach crunches should also be avoided.

And after my baby is delivered?

You should start your pelvic floor exercises as soon as possible, which will help prevent urinary incontinence. You can also do stretches and walking. Swimming may be resumed as soon as the bleeding has settled after the delivery of your baby. This is usually after about 2 weeks.

If you have had a Caesarean Section, you should check with your GP before you resume exercise, but you can immediately start on your pelvic floor exercises. You should take extra care and gradually resume high impact sports as the ligaments that have stretched during pregnancy can take some months to regain their previous strength.

Exercise after the birth of your baby will hasten the speed of your physical recovery, will help you lose your pregnancy weight gain (as will breast feeding) and will also help keep away post natal depression. Moderate exercise has no effect on the quality or quantity of breast milk you produce but make sure you drink plenty and you have adequate bust support while you exercise as your breasts may be quite tender.

What about exercising if I have a medical problem?

If you have a medical problem check with your GP before you start exercising as to what is suitable for you. There are Exercise Referral Schemes that your GP can refer you to. The idea of this is that your GP can prescribe a course of exercise that is specifically suited to your needs.

There is much evidence that exercise is beneficial for many medical problems. Exercise Referral Programmes can be gym based or can offer aerobics classes. Some swimming pools offer schemes and there are programmes such as "tea dancing" available in some areas.

The programme consists of an initial assessment of your base level of fitness and introduces from there a graded exercise programme, suited to your needs, lasting usually for 3 months.

This is available for adults of all ages with an extremely diverse range of medical problems from heart disease and high blood pressure to back pain, arthritis and depression. The schemes are run at a reduced cost to the patient. The programme should be the first step in teaching you how to manage your own exercise regime. The idea is that when the programme ends you continue your regime on your own.

Also available in many areas are free walking schemes run by the local council. The walks are guided group walks and free of charge and can be a great way to get fit while meeting like-minded people.

Ask your GP for information.

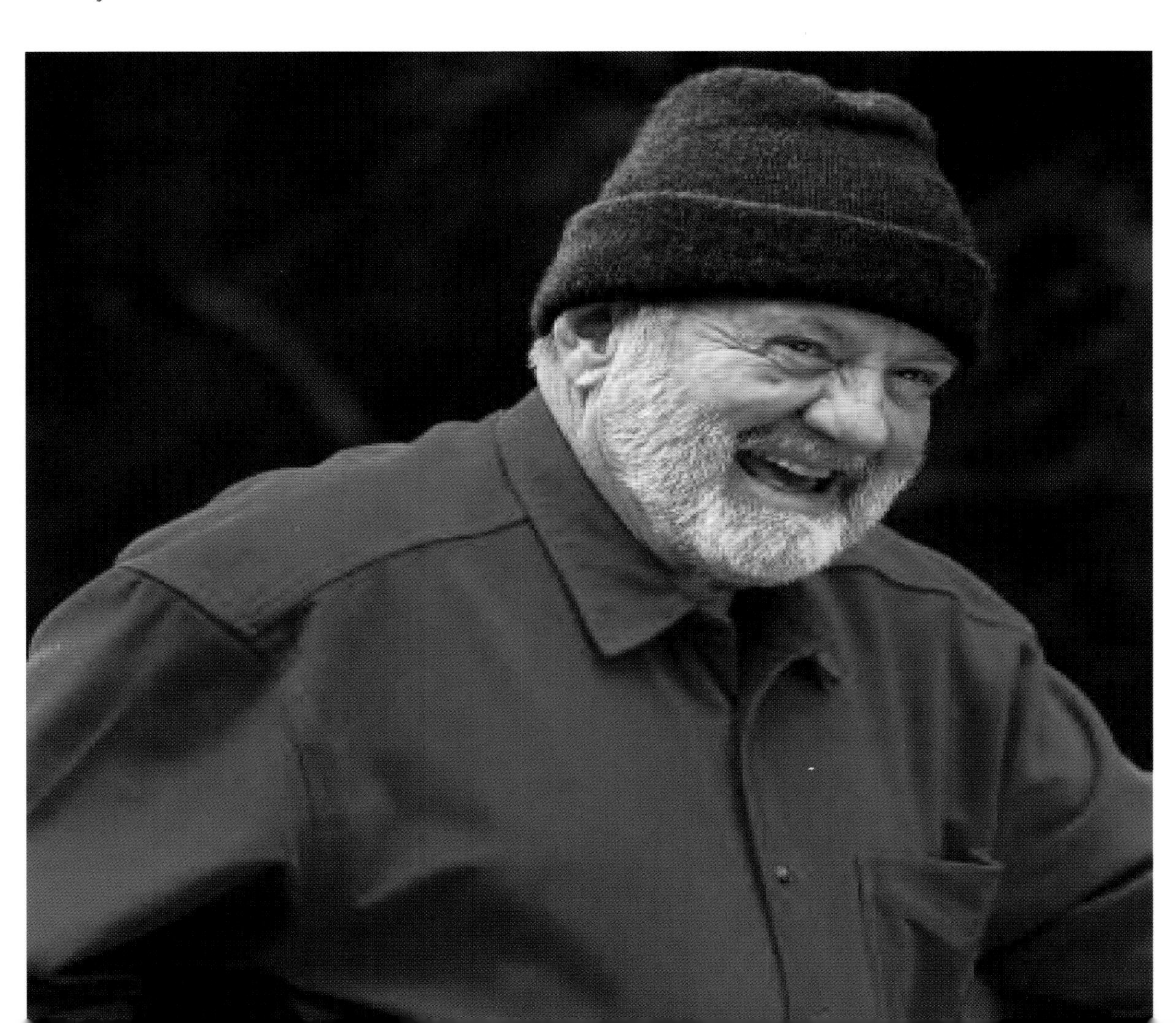

What if I have a heart problem?

If you have had a heart attack, your GP or your Cardiologist should refer you to a Cardiac Rehabilitation Programme. You should not give up exercising because you have had a heart attack. In fact the reverse is true. We positively encourage you to do regular exercise. This will rebuild strength in your heart and will help control your blood pressure and your blood cholesterol.

A Cardiac Rehabilitation Programme teaches you about your heart and how to look after it. It takes you through a graded exercise programme, gradually building up what you can do, under supervision. The aim is that you will finish the programme possibly fitter than before you had your heart attack and that continuing some form of exercise thereafter will help prevent a further heart attack.

If you have a heart condition make sure that you build up your exercise level gradually. Dress warmly in cold or windy weather as the cold can cause angina. Don't exercise on a full stomach. If you suffer with angina, make sure you always take your GTN spray with you and stop exercising if you get any pain or feel dizzy, excessively short of breath or sick.

What about if I have trouble breathing?

There are Pulmonary Rehabilitation Programmes available through your GP or local hospital if you suffer with chronic lung disease. These programmes take you through a 12 week exercise programme in addition to teaching you about your condition and how to best manage it. If you suffer with Emphysema or Chronic Bronchitis (smoker's lung), Pulmonary Rehabilitation has been shown to dramatically improve your quality of life, decrease admissions to hospital and has also been shown to halve the length of your stay if you are admitted as a result of your lung condition. Ask your GP for information.

What about if I have a disability?

Having a disability does not preclude you from exercise. In fact, it is more important that you do.

Take a look at the following web sites:
www.inclusivefitness.org

This site provides information on local gyms and sports facilities available for the disabled. The programme supports the fitness industry to make it more inclusive by increasing accessibility, equipment and staffing, and is designed to allow those with a disability to participate.

A neighbour of mine had a major stroke 2 years ago, leaving him wheelchair bound with the use of only one of his hands. This summer he abseiled, kayaked, sailed and did a zip wire through a local group, the Calvert Trust. Have a look at their web site on: www.calvert-trust.org.uk

This organisation has 3 centres throughout the UK and in addition to day activities also offers residential holidays. You can also contact them on: telephone: 01598 763 221

At my local pool a blind gentleman comes regularly and swims. He has a companion who tells him when to turn and the life guard ropes off a lane, so he can swim without colliding with other swimmers.

The National Centre of Physical Activity and Disability provides information, including books and videos on exercises you can do if you have disabilities, including disability following a stroke. Take a look on: www.ncpad.org

The Ramblers web site provides information for those who have a disability and would like to do some walking. Take a look on:
www.ramblers.org.uk/INFO/everyone/disability.html

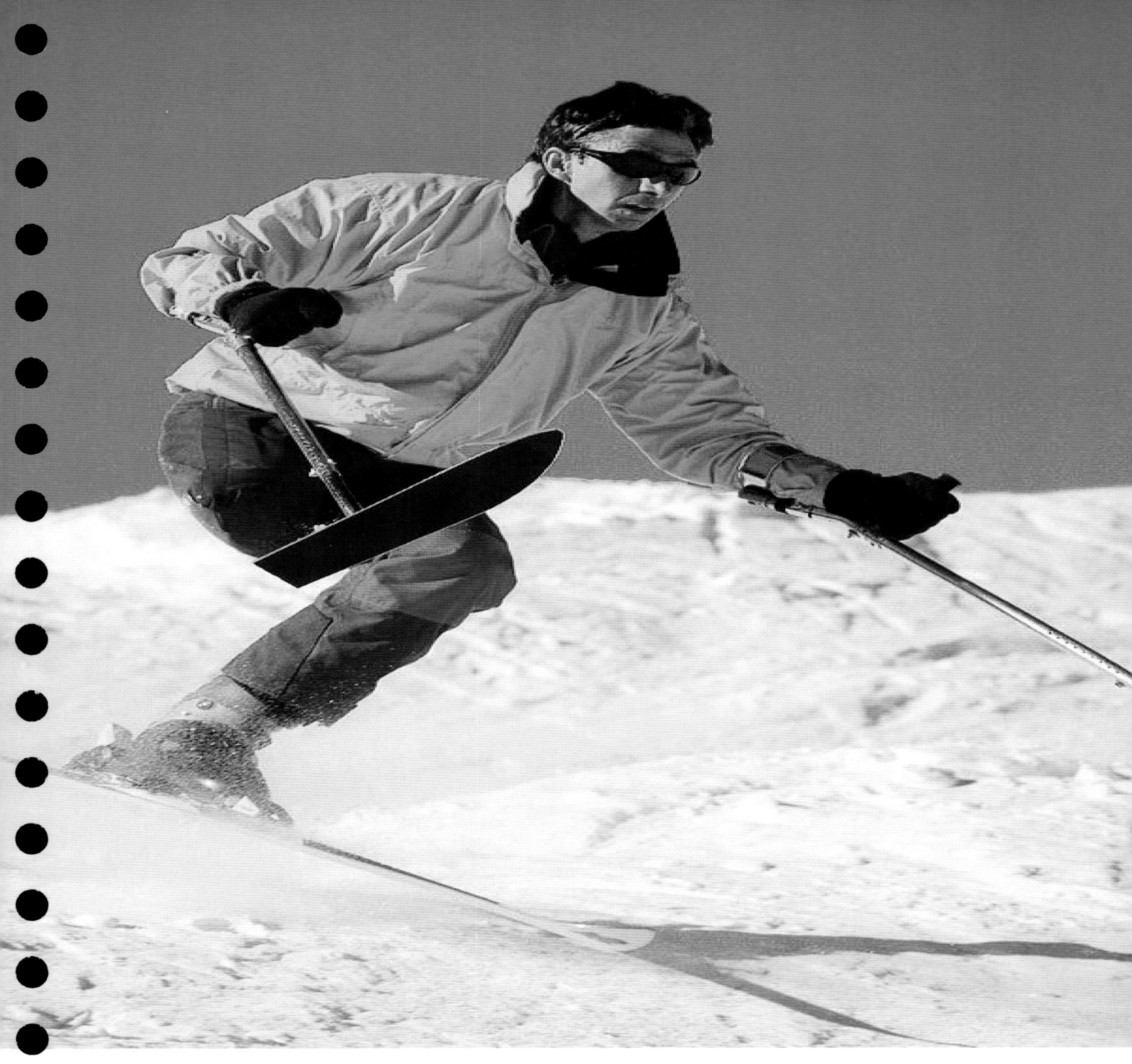

What if I'm a carer?

Many carers find it difficult to get out of the house to exercise when they have the 24 hour responsibility of looking after someone else. There are several National Organisations that provide carers with the opportunity to get out and have a break for whatever they want to do. This could be to do your shopping, get your hair done, to exercise or simply to sleep. Relief carers are fully trained. Contact your local Social Services for information. The services provided are means tested and cost depends on the level of care required. You can also contact: www.crossroads.org.uk
also available on telephone: 0845 450 0350

"You must be the change you wish to see in the world"

Mahatma Ghandi

What about exercising if I am too overweight?

Some people find that they are so overweight that they are unable to get started on even the most basic of exercise regimes. Others, that they are too embarrassed to go to the gym or to put on a swimming costume because of their size. Whatever your size, it is possible to exercise. Here are a few tips:

Consult your GP before starting exercising. Start gently and be prepared to build up gradually. It may be all that you can do when you start is walk to the corner of the road before getting breathless or tired.

Walking is a really good way to start. Many people who are overweight suffer with painful joints. Swimming or aqua-aerobics are beneficial, because the water supports your weight and so is kind to your joints. If you are worried about getting into the pool in a costume, check whether your local pool runs single sex sessions, or has times dedicated to groups who are overweight.

If you can't swim or lack water confidence, many pools run adult swimming lessons.

Have a look at: www.obesityservices.org

This company sell a DVD called "Weigh 2 Win" which is designed to give options of exercising to people who are very overweight, including chair exercise regimes.

Stay focused. Keep going. It may take you some time to get to fitness, but if you stick at it, you will succeed. Take a look at Part Two on "Make a healthy lifestyle change" for some ideas.

Myth:	Sit ups will get rid of the fat around your tummy.
Myth buster:	They won't. They will tone the muscle under the fat. When you exercise fat is lost gradually from all over the body.

What should I expect when I first start exercising?

How you feel after exercise will depend on how much or how vigorously you have exercised. If you build up gradually you should feel refreshed and probably a little tired. Many people feel inhibited about exercising before or after a long day at work because of the feeling of anticipated tiredness. The tiredness that you experience is not groggy but relaxed and as a result your brain ticks over more clearly. I find that I am far more productive at work if I have exercised beforehand and have far more, rather than less energy, in the evenings after an exercise session. I also find that my quality of sleep is better.

You might find that the muscles you have worked if unaccustomed to that level of exercise will be a little achy. This will be at its worst the following day and then will settle down. There is nothing wrong with this and you will find as you become accustomed to this level of exercise that it disappears.

Your muscles shouldn't be extremely painful; neither should your tendons (the tissues that connect your muscles to your bones) or joints. If you find that you have bad pain following exercise, check before you exercise next time, that you warm up and down properly, don't exercise too vigorously and that you are wearing the proper footwear or using the correct type or size equipment for your sport. If this persists, then consult your doctor.

You may find it takes a while to settle into a routine when you first start exercising, until your body becomes accustomed to the change in regime. In general, the more you do it, the easier it gets.

I find after I have exercised that I am far less stressed.

Rather than taking time out of my day, exercising creates time, because I have more energy in the evenings and so I am able to stay up later and the jobs that I do are done with greater efficiency and therefore more quickly.

It can take a while to get to a level where you feel like this. It's worth the wait. Believe me, the rewards are fantastic when you finally get there.

Try this today

Choose one thing and go for it. Have fun:

- Set out a treasure hunt in the park for your children
- Pump the tires up on your bicycle
- Walk the children home from school or go for a walk in your lunch break with a colleague
- Sign up for a new exercise class
- Get in the sea
- Kick a football around the garden with your children
- When you throw a ball for your dog, run after it too
- Get up early and go for a swim
- Go dancing

"Angels whisper to a man when he goes for a walk"

Raymond Inmon

How should I go about doing a good warm up and warm down?

A good warm up and warm down are designed to prevent injury and also to improve your flexibility, balance, co-ordination, mobility and strength. Warming up prepares you both mentally and physically for your exercise.

What you do to warm up will depend on what you intend to do for your exercise. The principles of a good warm up should be to increase blood flow around your body, which in turn decreases muscle stiffness and improves joint lubrication.

Your warm up should be a gentle and yet dynamic routine, specifically tailored to your chosen sport. Static stretching exercises, (that is stretching exercises in which you hold your stretch) should not be done to warm up.

If, for instance, your exercise is walking, you should simply start your walk more slowly and increase your speed after about 5-6 minutes, to a brisk walk.

If however you choose a more aerobic sport such as running, cycling, swimming, or a racquet sport, you should spend the first 5-6 minutes doing your chosen activity at a gentle pace. This should be followed by 5-10 minutes of dynamic stretches, specific to your sport. Sports using the lower limbs use dynamic stretches more focused on the legs, whereas sports using the upper limbs such as swimming focus more on the arms. Racquet sports need stretches for both.

Some simple dynamic stretches for your legs before jogging might be:

- a gentle jog, alternately bringing each knee up to ninety degrees

- slow jog, kicking your bottom with your feet

- skipping, springing off your toes, bringing your knees up high and working your arms to add to your momentum

For your arms and upper body before swimming or a racquet sport, a good warm up might be walking briskly while:

- circling your arms forwards

- circling your arms backwards

- holding your elbows at shoulder height, with your palms facing the floor and your elbows bent and bringing your elbows in an arc behind the line of your shoulders, keeping your arms bent and straightening them alternately (think Barbara Windsor in Carry On Camping!).

Your cool down is as important as your warm up and should involve 5-10 minutes at the end of your workout. You should start this with slowing down the pace of your chosen activity for 5 minutes. You should then spend 5-10 minutes doing static stretches.

The stretches you do should stretch the muscle groups you have used. Each stretch should be held initially for 15 seconds. At this point you will feel your muscle relax and you should gently increase the stretch for a further 10 seconds.

Don't bounce when you stretch. Hold each stretch gently and make sure you breathe throughout.

If you would like some ideas for static stretches, your local gym may be able to advise you.

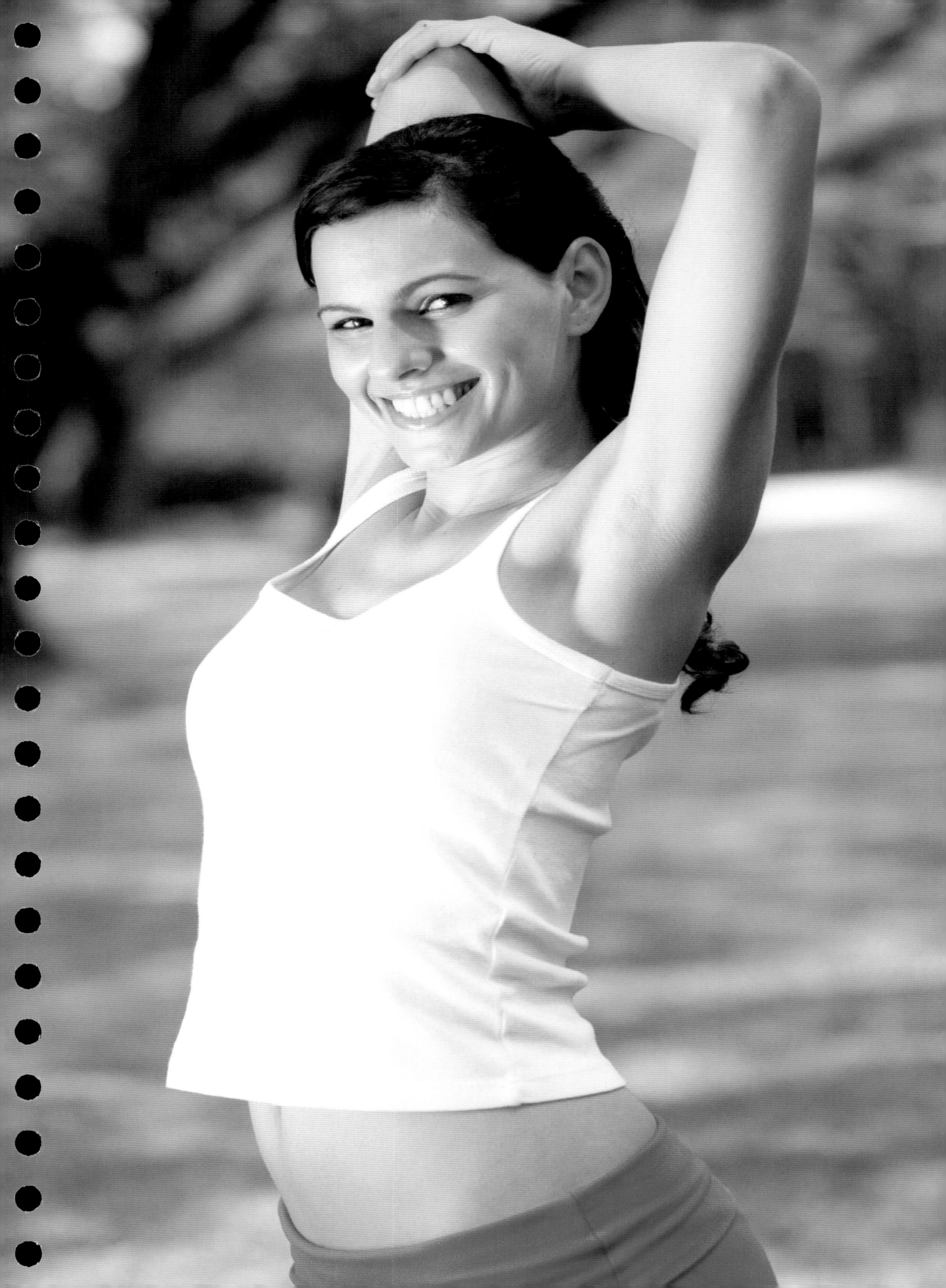

Paul's story

Paul is 45 years old and has been diagnosed with high blood pressure. He works in the city and commutes 1½ hours each way, setting off at 7am and getting home at around 8pm. He works through most lunch times in order to get his work finished. This is the norm within his office. In order to avoid the rush hour each night, he and a group of friends from work go to a local wine bar. There he drinks 3-4 glasses of wine over an hour or so before heading home.

Paul weighs 19kg (3 stone) over his ideal weight. He doesn't smoke and does no exercise, as there just isn't the time. He spends his weekends with his partner or with a group of good friends and loves watching any kind of sport on TV. He regularly drinks several cans of lager while doing so.

He feels irritated by the fact that he has been told by his GP that he needs to make some healthy life changes, but his father had high blood pressure and had a heart attack when he was in his 50s and he realises that he probably ought to do something about it.

Paul needs to lose weight, increase his exercise level and decrease his alcohol consumption (he is pleased to hear that a glass of wine a day is beneficial for his heart, but wonders how he will manage to achieve a day or 2 alcohol free a week).

Paul decides to get off the train a stop early once a week, on the only day that he has no fixed commitments in the morning. His working day is pushed later by half an hour, but he still manages to get one drink in with his friends before going home on the train! As he recognises that his motivation is poor he decides to ask a group of friends with whom he normally drinks to join a local sports club. On 3 days a week after work, instead of going to the wine bar, they exercise together, doing either, circuit training, a gym workout or 5 a side football. They still go for a drink afterwards together, but only have one, as most of them have to get back to partners or families.

At the weekend Paul and his partner go to their local gym together on a Saturday morning. He finds that having someone to exercise with, motivates him not only to get there, but to do well when he is there. His relationships with both his partner and his colleagues have improved as a result of the exercise that they do together. He still watches sport on TV for much of the weekend, but limits himself to a maximum of 2 cans of lager whilst doing so.

After 3 months Paul has lost 5kg (11lb), is less stressed at work, more alert in the evenings and is up for promotion. His blood pressure is still borderline, but does not require him to take any medication.

Encouraged by his success, he and his partner decide to embark on a healthy eating plan. As Paul's father had high cholesterol and his is on the high side, they decide to start by looking at cutting out some of the fats that they have in their diet. They swap from full fat to semi-skimmed milk, change from butter to margarine, and have a pasta meal on a Sunday rather than a roast.

My thoughts

I am really pleased with Paul's progress. The disadvantage at the outset with Paul was that his motivation was coming from an external source, that is, that he has been told by his GP that he needs to make some health changes. If your need to change comes from within, the impetus to change is far more powerful.

Paul's other limiting factor was time and a strong peer group who shared the same ethos of heavy drinking.

It was therefore important that he made changes in a way that would not only motivate him but would keep him going back for more.

The ways in which he achieved these things were:

- He prepared his foundations well by choosing exercise that he would enjoy and building it into his life so that it became an integral part of both his home and work life.

- He chose exercise in several different forms, which made his involvement varied, interesting and above all fun. Another way of motivating himself might have been to choose a form of exercise which involved a goal of some sort. For instance jogging with a goal of building up to a particular running event, such as a local fun run or swimming with the aim of getting involved in an event like the annual "swimathon," a UK national sponsored swimming event (see www.swimathon.org).

- He starts by setting himself several small achievable goals and builds on them gradually. He keeps his expectations realistic.

- He takes control of what goals he sets and at what time, rather than working to another's agenda.

- He engages the support of friends and family, by getting them to exercise with him. This in itself is a form of reward, in terms of what you achieve in the bonds of friendship made through exercise.

- He thinks long term. After 3 months he has made good progress, but still leads a far from perfect health life. He doesn't rush to achieve all at once, but paces himself well.

Exercise
(One small step for man; one giant leap for mankind)

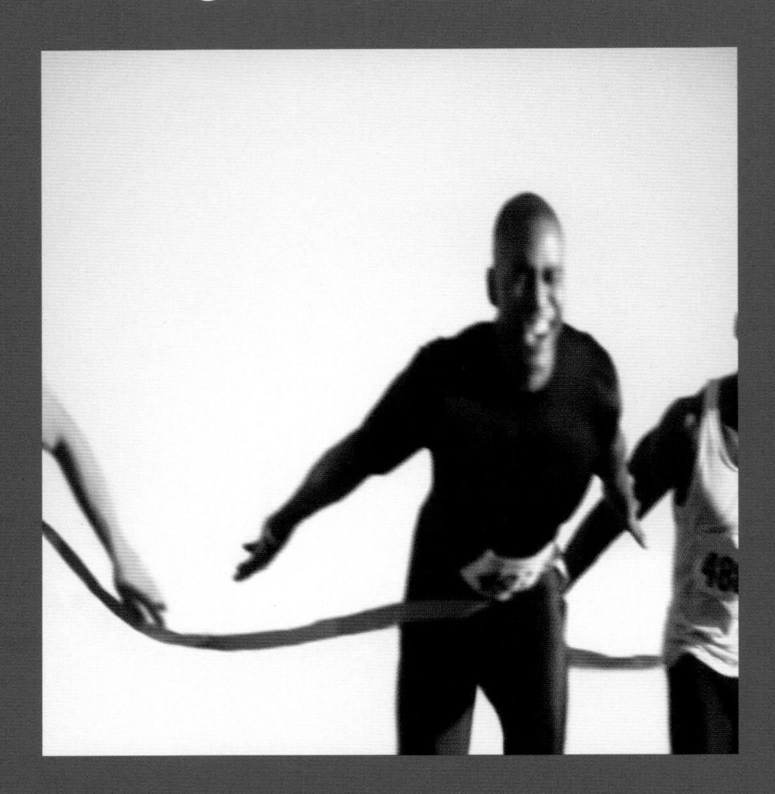

Remember

- The recommended level of exercise is 30 minutes, 5 times a week
- Any exercise is better than none
- Choose something that you enjoy
- Get involved with more than one type of exercise
- Build up gradually
- Most medical conditions benefit from exercise

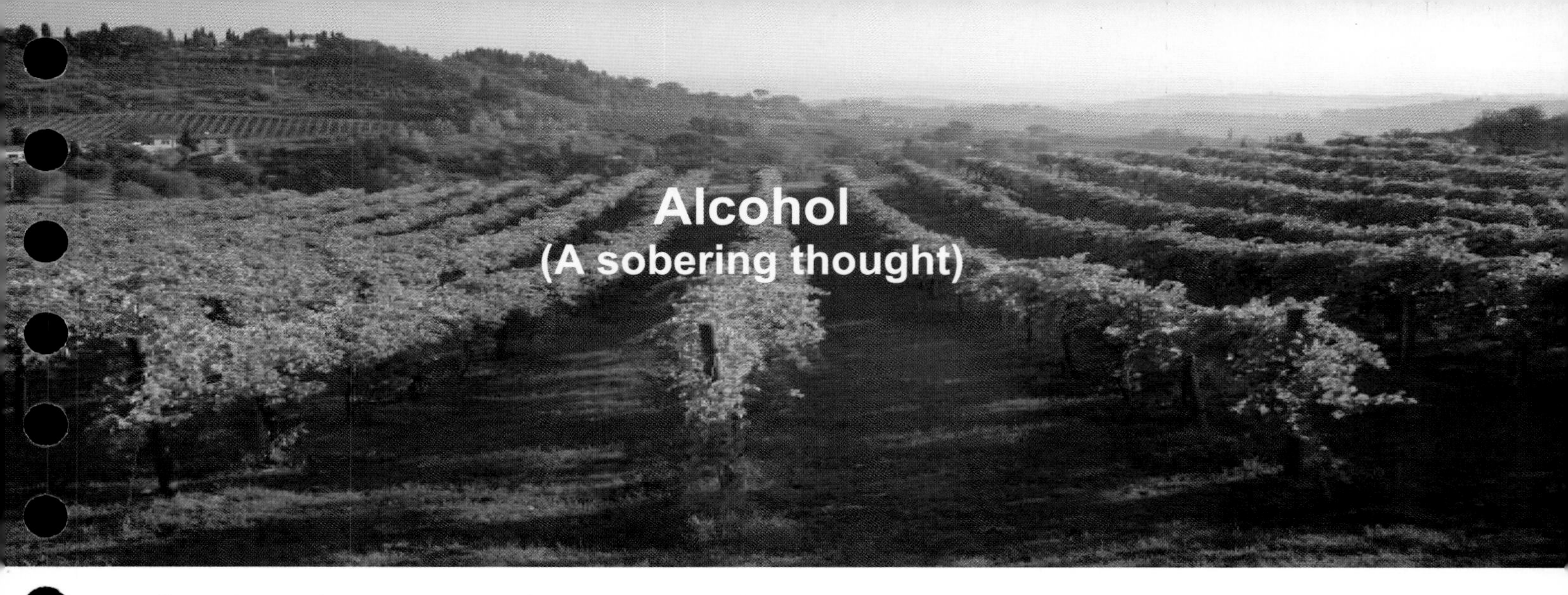

Alcohol
(A sobering thought)

I've always been a glass of wine a night girl. No more, no less; but nevertheless every night. It came as quite a shock a few years ago, when I thought that I would try to stop for a couple of months to "see what would happen" and I was unable to do so (at least on the first attempt anyway). I have to say I listened with interest to the latest figures that show that the group who drink the most in the UK are middle class women.

The level of alcohol misuse is increasing in the UK. In 2005 over a third of men and a quarter of women were found to be drinking over the safe limit of alcohol, with one in nine men being dependent on alcohol. There has been a worrying increase in the number of people in their twenties and thirties being treated for liver failure, as a result of alcohol misuse at a young age.

Of equal concern is the fact that alcohol use is increasing in children. Alcohol concern published figures in 2006 to show that 54% of 11-15 year olds use alcohol. This number has decreased to date, but latest figures show that although the number of children drinking has gone down, the amount of alcohol that the ones who do drink, has increased.

My daughter is 11 years old and the thought of what lies ahead in her teenage years in this climate of heavy drinking terrifies me.

The recommended safe upper limit of alcohol consumption for adults in the UK is 21 units a week for men and 14 units a week for women

Women are affected more by alcohol than men which is why their safe limit is lower. It is particularly worrying therefore that the greatest increase in heavy drinking is amongst women.

Home units, (the glass you pour for yourself) tend to be larger than pub measures, so be careful if you drink regularly at home.

A good guide is to have no more than 2 units a day if you are a woman and no more than 3 units a day if you are a man. Always try and have 2 or 3 days alcohol free a week if possible.

Myth:	Alcohol lifts mood and makes you feel better
Myth buster:	Alcohol disinhibits behaviour but in fact lowers mood. Drinking too much can lead to depression

What is a unit?

Everyone seems to have a different idea of what constitutes a unit. Wine can vary in strength from bottle to bottle and it is partly because there has been an increase in bottle strength over the last few years that confusion has arisen.

You can calculate the number of units in a glass by multiplying the volume in litres by the percentage alcohol: A standard pub measure (125 ml) of a small glass of wine (12% alcohol by volume) contains 1.5units.

0.125 L x 12% = 1.5 units

A ½ pint (287ml) of lager, cider or beer (3-4% alcohol by volume)= 1 unit.

A standard single pub measure (25 ml) spirit
(40% alcohol by volume)= 1 unit.

A standard pub measure (50ml) glass sherry/ port
(20% alcohol by volume)= 1 unit.

Please note:

Strong beer (6% alcohol by volume) contains 6 units in one litre, so 1 pint (575 ml) contains just over 3 units.

Alcohol consumption may increase your risk of breast cancer

"If drinking is interfering with your work, you're probably a heavy drinker. If work is interfering with your drinking, you're probably an alcoholic"

Author unknown

What is binge drinking?

Binge drinking is drinking too much over a short period of time. There is no internationally agreed definition of what constitutes binge drinking but drinking surveys in the UK normally define it as drinking 8 units or more for men and 6 units or more for women.

40% of all drinking is done as binge drinking in the UK. This is most common in the 16-24 age group. Binge drinking increases your risk of accidents, violent incidents and unsafe sex.

What are the risks of drinking too much alcohol?

Increase in cancers: this includes cancer of the mouth, pharynx, larynx, oesophagus and liver. There is also a link with breast cancer and cancer of the rectum.

Increase in liver cirrhosis and liver failure: with the rise in heavy drinking in young people, there has been a dramatic increase in the number of people in their twenties and thirties suffering with liver failure.

Increase in other medical problems: stomach ulcers, pancreatitis, high blood pressure, strokes, memory loss, sexual difficulties and vitamin deficiencies.

Increase in accidents: in 2005, 15,000 people were killed or injured in drink driving accidents.

Increase in mental illness: alcohol is a depressant and can worsen or cause depression. Alcohol can increase levels of aggression. 65% of suicides are linked with excess drinking.

Increase in crime: 66% of male sentenced prisoners and 80% of female sentenced prisoners admit to hazardous drinking in the months prior to imprisonment.

Increase in unsafe sex: the risk of rape, assault or unsafe sex increases with heavy drinking.

Are there benefits to alcohol?

The good news is that once you hit middle age (age 44 in men and after the menopause in women) that drinking a small to moderate amount of alcohol can reduce your risk of heart disease.
This is more pronounced in men than women, simply because men are at greater risk of heart disease. Until middle age, your risks of drinking alcohol outweigh the benefits.

Research shows that all alcohol carries that protective benefit, however red wine seems to give the greatest protection.

Even at middle age and above, it is important to have one or two alcohol free days a week.

Why should I cut down on my alcohol consumption?

If you drink over the recommended safe upper limit of alcohol per week the chances are that your body is suffering. If you have done this for a long period of time, you may well have forgotten what it is like to feel great.

Cutting down or stopping alcohol consumption will have benefits in many areas.

You will reduce the risk of all the aforementioned problems. In addition some of the immediate benefits include: You will wake in the morning feeling refreshed from good quality sleep. Your snoring will improve. You will have a clear head. Your thinking and reasoning will be improved. Your mood will lift and you will feel less aggressive. Your relationships at work and home will strengthen. Your sugar cravings and headaches will lessen; your skin will clear and you will lose weight. Constipation will improve and drinking less alcohol can even improve urinary incontinence.

Now is the time to act. Make a resolution to make a change today.

Drinking and Driving

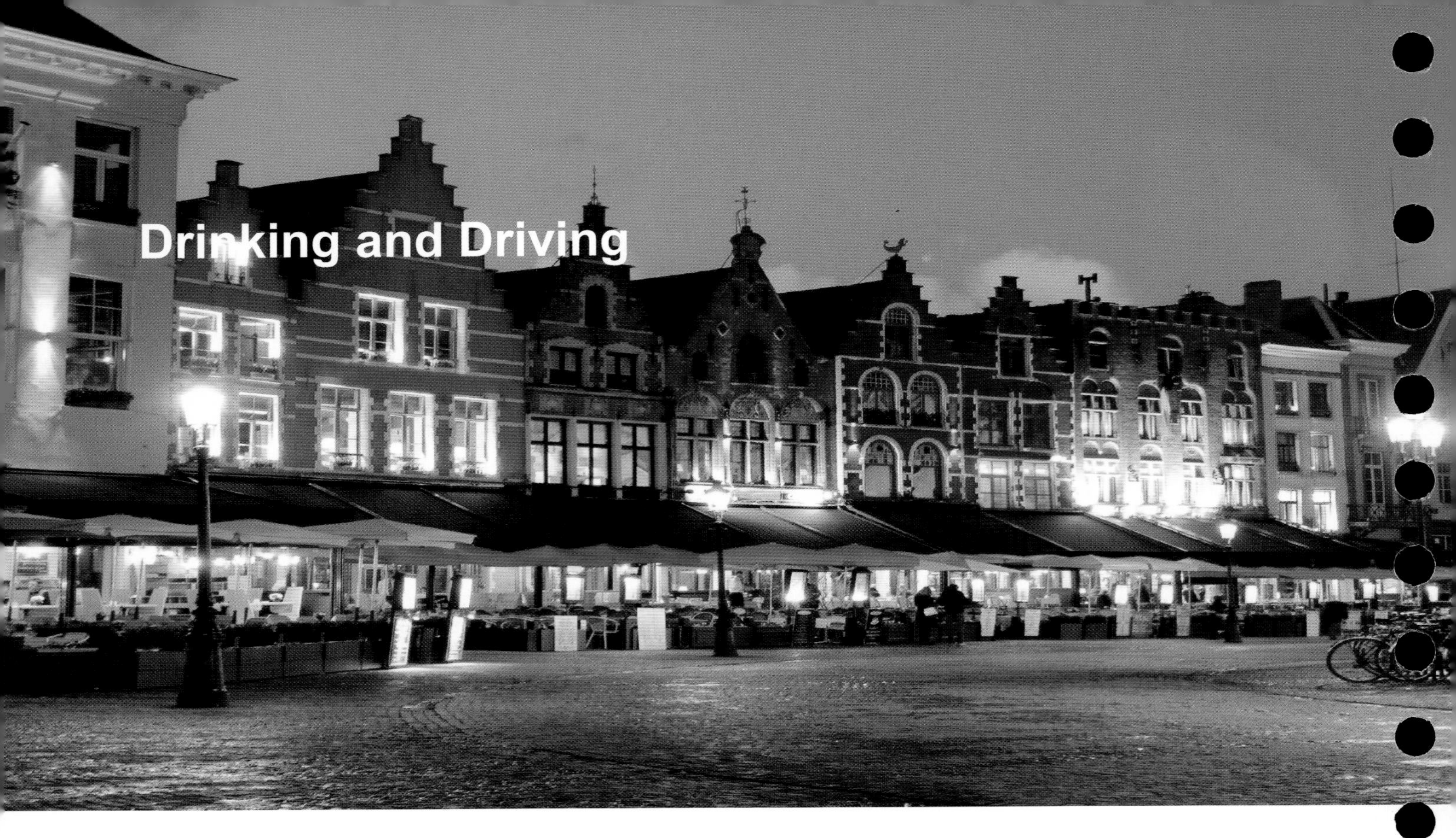

The legal limit for driving is 80mg of alcohol in 100ml blood. There is a general misconception about how much is safe to drink and drive. Many people think that "a couple" of drinks will be OK. Everyone's body handles alcohol slightly differently, so there is no way of telling when you have got to your legal limit. It is therefore impossible to translate this figure into how many pints of beer or glasses of wine or spirits you can have.

Your safe limit tends to be lower if you are a woman; young, slim and you haven't eaten. It can also depend on the type of drink that you are drinking. Certain medications can also affect your driving ability.

If you have been drinking heavily the night before, you may still be over the limit in the morning and therefore unsafe to drive.

> Beth's top tip:
> Even if you have not reached your legal upper limit, your driving ability is affected. If you are breathalysed and the police officer thinks that your driving was influenced by alcohol, you can be prosecuted regardless.

The only way to be absolutely sure is not to drink at all if you are going to drive.

Myth:	Beer contains less alcohol than spirits.
Myth buster:	½ a pint (287ml) of beer contains the same amount of alcohol as a single measure of spirits.

Can I drink when I am pregnant?

Drinking alcohol to excess during pregnancy, can cause a condition called Foetal Alcohol Syndrome (FAS). This consists of poor growth of the baby with central nervous system defects, lowered IQ and facial malformations.

There is confusing advice being given by different agencies at the moment which makes it very difficult for women to know which path to follow as to what is the safe upper limit for alcohol consumption in pregnancy.

The National Institute for Clinical Excellence (NICE) issued guidance in 2007 that women should limit themselves to less than one standard drink (1.5 units or 12g alcohol) per day during pregnancy and to avoid it completely during the first three months.

The Department of Health brought out guidance saying that women should avoid alcohol altogether during pregnancy.

There is conflicting advice simply because at the moment, we are not sure. There is no convincing evidence that drinking a small amount of alcohol in pregnancy is harmful to your unborn child, but we can't completely exclude the possibility.

For this reason, until we are sure, the sensible thing to do is to avoid alcohol through your pregnancy.

Myth:	If you drink lots of water before going to bed when you have had a heavy night drinking, you will be fine.
Myth buster:	Water prevents dehydration caused by alcohol and so helps you feel less hung over the morning but it doesn't prevent your liver being damaged by the alcohol you consume.

How do I cut down on my drinking?

Set a target

Use the guideline of the recommended safe limits on page 61 to work out how much alcohol you want to drink in a week. Specify how many days you want to keep alcohol free and on days when you are drinking, how much you want to drink as your upper limit.

Keep an alcohol diary

Record all the alcoholic drinks you consume over the course of a week. Record who you are with when you drink and what you were doing at the time. You will build up a good idea of your drinking pattern and your triggers (that is what makes you want to drink), from this exercise. It's really important to be honest with yourself. Remember to include drinks that you have during the day as well as your evening drinks.

Refer to the Personal Health Plan at the back of the book. Page 140 is dedicated to your Alcohol Diary with some more hints as to how you might go about filling it in.

Make a plan

Using the knowledge that you have gained from your Alcohol Diary, plan some strategies that you can use to reduce your alcohol consumption. You need to recognise your weaknesses and triggers and to put in place a strategy that will help you conquer each of them. Look at "safety netting" on page 118 for some ideas and record them on your "Alcohol Triggers" page in your Personal Health Plan on page 141. There are some exercises in Part Two, "Make a permanent healthy lifestyle change" (pages 85-128) which should help. These include visualisation, positive thinking, goal setting, safety netting and reward.

Stay motivated

Make a list of the ways in which you will benefit from cutting down on your drinking levels. You can pin this to the fridge or carry it around with you. Keep looking at it. Use the visualisation techniques described on page 86 to keep these positive images in your mind. Write down your ideas on page 141 of your Personal Health Plan.

Enlist support

Get your partner or a friend on board. In particular if you drink in a group, it is really useful to have another member of that group helping you. Your GP will be able to offer you advice. Call the help-lines mentioned later in this section. They provide a free service with trained counsellors.

Be good to yourself

If you slip up, don't beat yourself up. Many people will have set backs. Guilt serves no purpose and in fact can be really destructive as it can deter you from trying again. Pick yourself up and review your plan. Make a note of how the knock occurred and put in place a strategy that will prevent it happening on a second occasion.

Reward your success

All successes deserve a reward. Have a look at some ideas on page 128 to plan how you might go about doing this, then record them on page 156.

What if I can't cut down on the amount I drink by myself?

Your GP will be able to give you advice regarding organisations that can help you. There are counsellors available both on the NHS and privately. NHS funding for residential inpatient detoxification is poor in some areas, except in more complex cases and so many areas now offer community detoxification programmes, with intensive support and follow up in the home.

For advice and information regarding alcohol you could contact Alcohol Concern at www.alcoholconcern.org.uk

64 Leman Street,
London,
E1 8EU.
telephone 0207 264 0510

Or Alcoholics Anonymous at www.alcoholics-anonymous.org.uk
telephone 0845 769 7555

Are there any medications that will help me stop drinking?

Disulfiram is a drug which is only available on prescription and is used to help in the treatment of patients with alcohol dependence. Some areas require you to be under the care of an alcohol specialist to obtain it while in other areas you might find that your GP can prescribe it.

It works by producing a set of particularly unpleasant side effects if you drink any alcohol while taking it. Symptoms you could experience might be, severe headache, nausea, breathlessness, palpitations, a feeling of pressure in the chest, and collapse.

Acamprosate is a drug used to help you maintain abstinence once you have stopped drinking. It acts by reducing the cravings for alcohol. It can be used for up to a year after you have stopped drinking. Possible side effects might be tummy upsets abdominal pain and skin rashes.

"An alcoholic has been lightly defined as a man who drinks more than his own Doctor"

Alvan L. Barach

Gemma's story

Gemma is 23 years old and went to see her GP because she blacked out after a heavy drinking session at a party and can't remember much of the evening in the lead up to the blackout. She drinks with a group of girls, going out every weekend and also on a Thursday night. They regularly drink 7-8 glasses of wine or bottles of Alcopop in an evening and on one of the weekend nights she would consume 3 or 4 shots of spirit in addition.

Gemma smokes 10 cigarettes a day and lives on ready meals as she never learnt to cook when living at home and has no inclination to learn now. She used to play hockey and run when she was at school, but has done nothing since she left. She does walk a brisk 10 minutes to the bus stop every day on her way to and from work.

Gemma was surprised to hear that she was well over the safe upper limit for alcohol consumption for women, of 14 units per week. She said that she would find it easy to keep a few days alcohol free as she did that already, but that it would be hard to cut down on the number of drinks she had on the nights where she was drinking as her friends really enjoyed a drink. She was aware that smoking was bad for her and expressed some desire to give up, but was not wholehearted in her commitment.

Incentives: Gemma has been saving money to go on holiday to Turkey with friends next year, but has been making little headway. We calculated that she was spending around £70 a week on alcohol and cigarettes. She decided that cutting down to the safe limit and stopping smoking would be a good way to save money and that she would put the money saved into a jar, as her "Turkey fund." She was pleased to hear that her walk to the bus stop counted towards a large part of her recommended weekly exercise level.

Following this Gemma decided that she needed to limit her nights out to the weekend and to cut down the number of drinks she had on those nights to 4 drinks a night. Her alcohol triggers were that particular group of friends, as when she was not with them, she had no particular desire to drink.

Gemma exchanged her weeknight out drinking, with a night out with a friend from that group, doing a short run. They decided to train for "The Race for Life" (a UK national sponsored fun run for women to raise money for Cancer Research UK) together as it was 3 miles long and they thought they could comfortably build up to this. They found that there was a training regime especially for beginners, to accompany the race, which they accessed via the internet and they enjoyed the running so much that they ended up going 3 times a week.

Gemma found that she was coughing when she ran and so tried to cut down on the amount that she was smoking, but gave up because she found it too hard to do on her own.

On her nights out with the girls, Gemma made sure she ate before she went, to limit the effects of the alcohol. When ordering spirits, she had been previously ordering doubles, so she found it easy to cut these down to singles, while appearing to keep pace with her friends. Similarly she would order a small rather than a large glass of wine. She found the occasional low alcohol lager during an evening was a good substitute for an Alcopop, as she was still holding a bottle and this almost felt like a "real "drink to her. When she went to parties she would make sure that she didn't top up her glass of wine, so that she could keep track of what she was drinking.

Following successfully finishing the Race for Life, Gemma and her friend phoned the NHS Smoking Quitline and set a date for giving up smoking.

My thoughts

Gemma's motivation for her visit to her GP was really powerful. Having blacked out and no memory of a large portion of the previous evening, she had great concern about what might have happened in her "blank hours."

The Advisory Council on the Misuse of Drugs published a report in 2007 which found that the most common weapon used in drug facilitated sexual assault was alcohol.

Gemma's strength lies in her motivation. Her potential limiting factors are her peer group.

Gemma is young. She has no partner. She has a job, which she doesn't particularly enjoy. Her friends therefore are her all. The power of her group of friends is huge. She needs to be one of the gang, to be accepted and to be having fun.

It is therefore really important that she works with this group, rather than against them.

Our approach needs to involve her friends and it needs to be fun.

Gemma's reward in the form of a holiday with her friends is also a strong motivating factor, as it reinforces her desire to succeed and keeps her focus going at the start, when building the routine into your life can be the most challenging.

Gemma finds confidence in her success in one area. There is a danger that having "failed" in her attempt to stop smoking that she gives up with all her good work. The self esteem that she has achieved from successfully tackling her drinking gives her the impetus she needs to continue.

She set herself a difficult goal, in "going it alone" in her quit smoking attempt. Having previously discussed safety netting ideas (take a look in the next section of the book for more ideas), she was prepared. We talked about this in terms of an inevitable challenge rather than failure. As a result, having given herself the time to recharge her strength of purpose, she was able to make plans to try again.

Alcohol
(A sobering thought)

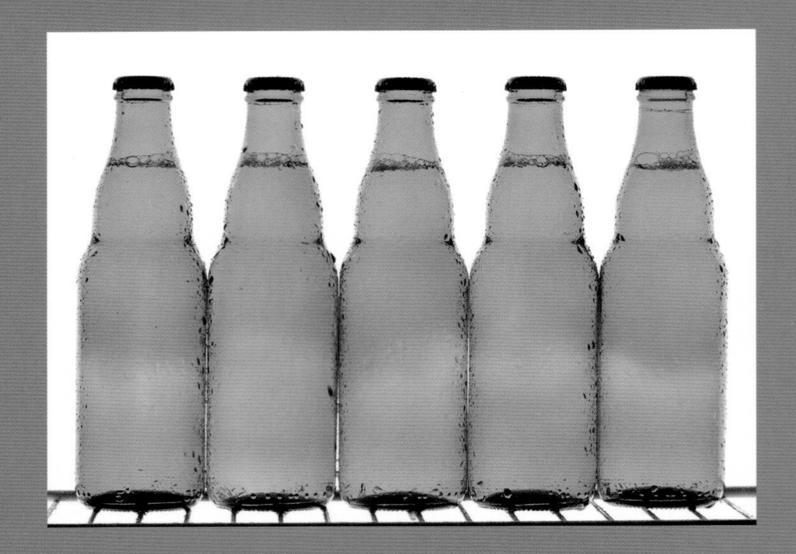

Remember

- Stick to your safe limits
- Watch your limits more closely if you are young, slim, haven't eaten, are driving or operating machinery
- Have 2-3 alcohol free days per week
- Avoid binge drinking
- Your driving ability will be affected even with a small amount of alcohol: don't drink and drive
- Avoid alcohol during pregnancy
- If you realise that you are dependent on alcohol, ask for help, before your health is permanently affected

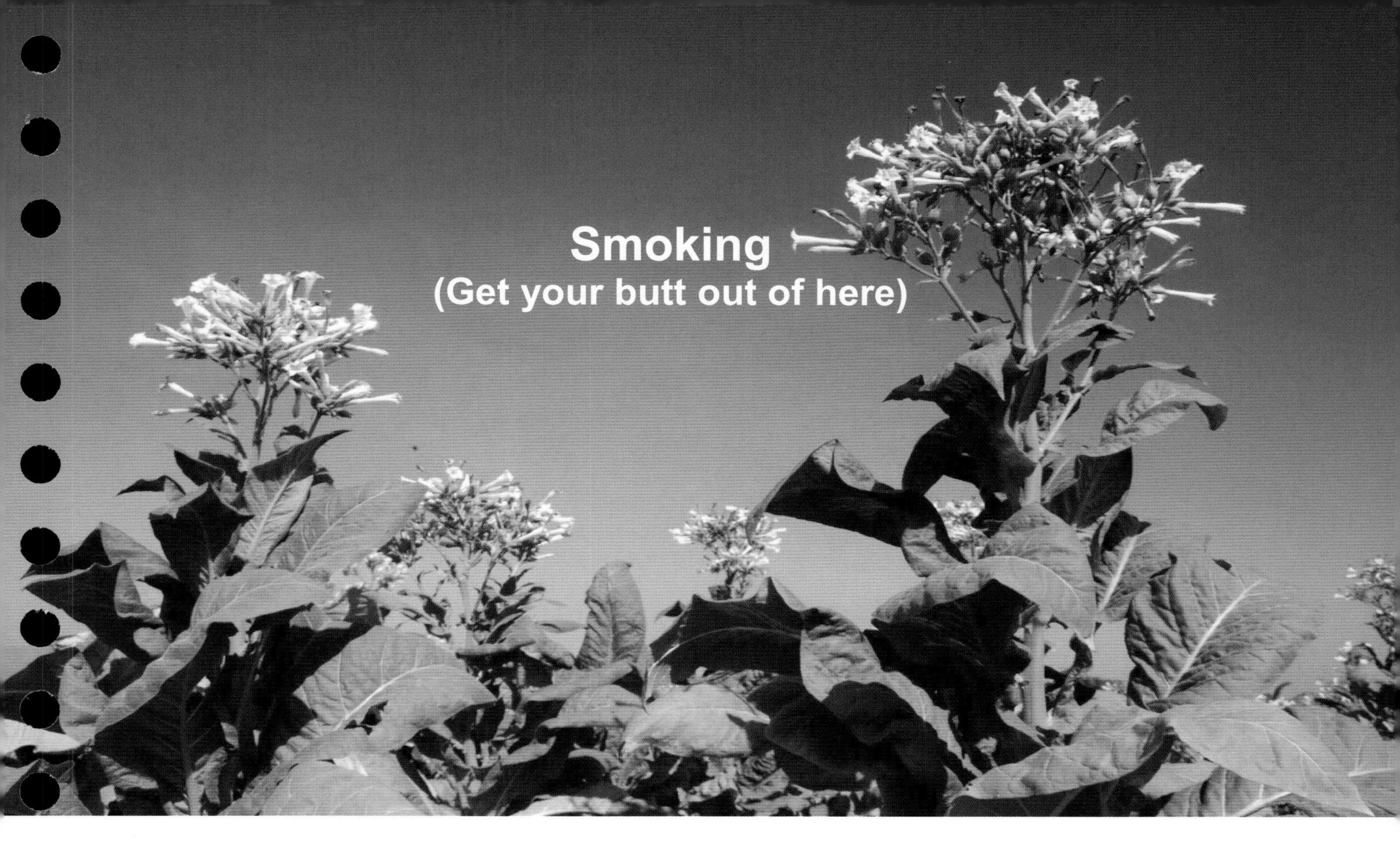

Smoking
(Get your butt out of here)

A friend of mine came to stay some time ago and when my son found her smoking in the garden, he told her that she shouldn't smoke because it was bad for her. She replied by throwing her cigarettes in the bin. My son couldn't work out why the next time she came to stay he found her smoking in the garden again. Mark Twain would have understood.

Smoking is the single greatest cause of ill health and death in the UK. There are 11 million regular smokers in Britain. 120,000 of these will die each year from smoking related illnesses, compared to 5,000 who die in road accidents.

The National Institute for Clinical Excellence (NICE) published figures in 2005 to say that the predicted decrease in life expectancy of smokers under the age of 35 years, if they continue to smoke, is 8 years. This does not take into account the reduction in quality of life due to stroke, heart and lung disease in the years leading up to death. Half of all smokers die prematurely from a smoking related illness.

The children of smokers are 2-3 times more likely to become smokers themselves. A child who has one parent who smokes inhales the equivalent of 50 cigarettes a year and if both parents smoke, this increases to 80. The number of children actively smoking has gone up despite Government Health of the Nation targets to reduce the level in this group.

Quitting at any age has immediate and long lasting benefit. If you manage to quit before the age of 35 years, you will have a life expectancy only slightly less than that of someone who has never smoked. Smokers halve their risk of heart attack within a year of stopping smoking.

"To stop smoking is the easiest thing I ever did; I ought to know because I've done it a thousand times"

Mark Twain

Why are cigarettes dangerous?

Cigarettes contain 3 main substances that cause the body harm: tar, carbon monoxide and nicotine.

Tar is the main disease forming element. It contains 4,000 chemicals and over 50 known carcinogens (cancer forming agents) and metabolic poisons. It is this that is responsible for lung cancers and bronchitis and emphysema (smoker's lung).

Carbon monoxide is a poisonous gas. When you inhale it while smoking, it inhibits the ability of your red blood cells to carry oxygen by up to about 15%. This means that your lungs work less efficiently. It is especially harmful during pregnancy as it reduces the amount of oxygen available to your baby for its healthy growth.

Nicotine is a substance with a powerful addictive capacity and is what causes problems with withdrawal symptoms when smokers are trying to quit. The mainstay of help with withdrawal symptoms, during your attempt to quit is therefore with nicotine replacement products or with products such as Bupropion Hydrochloride and Varenicline which block the nicotine receptors in the body so that you gain no pleasure from the nicotine when you smoke.

A smoker of 20 a day, spends over £2,000 a year on cigarettes

Myth:	**Smoking low tar or filtered cigarettes is OK**
Myth buster:	**A filter doesn't stop many of the cancer forming agents reaching your lungs. People who smoke these kinds of cigarette tend to inhale more deeply and more frequently with each cigarette.**

What diseases are caused by smoking?

Cancers: lung, mouth, nose and throat, larynx, oesophagus, pancreas, stomach, bladder, kidney, and leukaemia.

Heart disease: angina and heart attacks. Peripheral arterial disease which causes blockage of the arteries to the limbs resulting in gangrene and amputations.

Respiratory disease: lung cancer, chronic bronchitis and emphysema, asthma, and recurrent chest infections.

What about passive smoking?

The government recently changed the laws regarding smoking in enclosed public places on the back of evidence that proves that passive smoking can damage your health. This includes a 10-30% increase in lung cancers to those who are under prolonged exposure.

And smoking in pregnancy?

Women who smoke during pregnancy have an increased risk of miscarriage and premature birth. Their babies tend to be smaller and grow more slowly. They also have an increased rate of cot death, asthma and glue ear and tend to be off school more and admitted into hospital more than other children.

Nicotine replacement therapy can be used during pregnancy, so please ask your GP if you would like some help.

Alternatively you can call:

NHS Pregnancy Smoking Helpline: 0800 169 9169

The benefits of giving up smoking

If you are a smoker of cigarettes, cigars or a pipe, stopping smoking is the single most beneficial thing that you will ever do in your life to improve your health

You will:

- reduce your risk of heart attack, stroke and high blood pressure
- reduce your risk of lung and other cancers
- be able to taste and smell better
- have fresher breath
- feel your breathing improve
- have fewer chest infections
- feel better in yourself
- improve the health of those around you, including your children
- save money
- look younger for longer, as smoking ages your skin and hair

How do I go about quitting smoking?

Get motivated

The most important factor in the process is your motivation. If you do not want to give up, you will find it far more difficult a process. You may want to give up smoking because you are pregnant, it may be because you, or a friend or relative have had a health scare or just because it is something that you have wanted to do for a long time. It doesn't matter what your motivation is, as long as it is there. If you are not ready at this point in time it may be better to work on your motivation until you are, before you start trying.

Once you have established that *you* really want to, you will need to emotionally psyche yourself up. I will give you the tools you need to tackle this with ease; visualisation, positive thinking and goal setting.

Set yourself a deadline

When embarking on healthy eating and exercise patterns it is sensible to start slowly and build up. The smoking story is slightly different. When attempting to quit smoking, there is lots of evidence to show that working at stopping smoking gradually is far less successful than stopping to a deadline.

You will find that the smoking cessation clinics will advocate setting yourself a dead-line and stopping on that day. This is simply because most people are more successful in their attempt to quit, that way. You will probably fall into that category

Use all resources available to you

Make use of all the resources that are available to you. You wouldn't go into an operation without an anaesthetic. Why disadvantage yourself at the outset of what is likely to be a challenging process anyway. Go the path that is well trodden and shown to have the best quit rates.

Myth:	Smoking lifts your mood.
Myth buster:	Research shows that teenage smokers are four times more likely to be depressed than non smokers

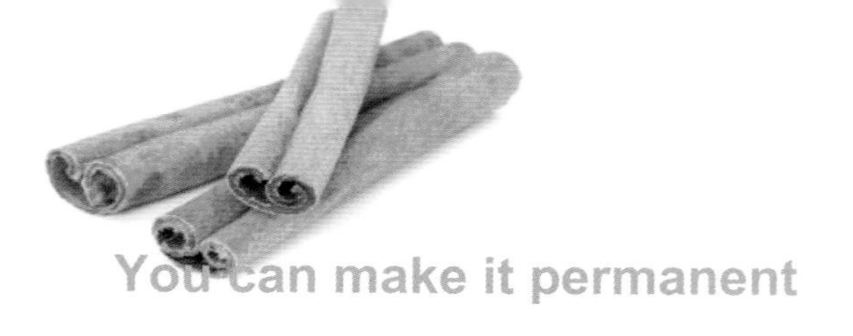

You can make it permanent

How you plan can make the difference between an unsuccessful or successful quit attempt. It's a bit like organising a holiday. You're much more likely to have a successful trip if you have thought ahead, planned an itinerary and what to take than, if you haven't. In not planning, you might still have a great holiday, but there's an equal chance you could end up with a suitcase full of nothing but underwear and nowhere to stay.

In the same way you should prepare in the lead up to your quit day.

Plan ahead and get your friends and family on board. Arrange something to do on the day you stop. This should be something that will keep you busy and is a change of routine. Make sure you spend the day with someone close to you, who is a non smoker and who is on board with your giving up smoking. Throw away all your cigarettes and empty all your ash trays, both in the car and house.

Make sure that you have any medication such as nicotine replacement products with you and that you have the Quit Line numbers to hand. Get a supply of carrots or celery sticks in the house to nibble on.

Many people only get this far in their heads in the lead up to their stop smoking dead line. You need to take this one step further. If in addition, you look forward, beyond your quit date and have some ideas for how you are going to keep things going beyond the initial few days, you are far more likely to succeed.

The section of this book, "Make a permanent healthy lifestyle change" will give you plenty of ideas. It shows you how to plan your goal, using positive thinking and deep relaxation techniques to aid you. Safety netting is a really good way of foreseeing problems before they arise and putting in place a strategy to cope to ensure that you are not set back. Visualisation techniques can also help to practice those situations in your head, before they occur, so that you are ready if or when they arise.

Your Personal Health Plan is at the back of the book and has a section to help you through your quit attempt. You can record your triggers for smoking and then can write down your ideas as to how you are going to overcome them (see page 143). Your smoking advisor (GP, Stop Smoking Clinic, chemist, quit-line or web site) should also be able to give you plenty of advice.

Try and capitalise on your success and start a healthy eating plan in combination with an exercise regime. This will help you keep any weight off and will help you feel great.

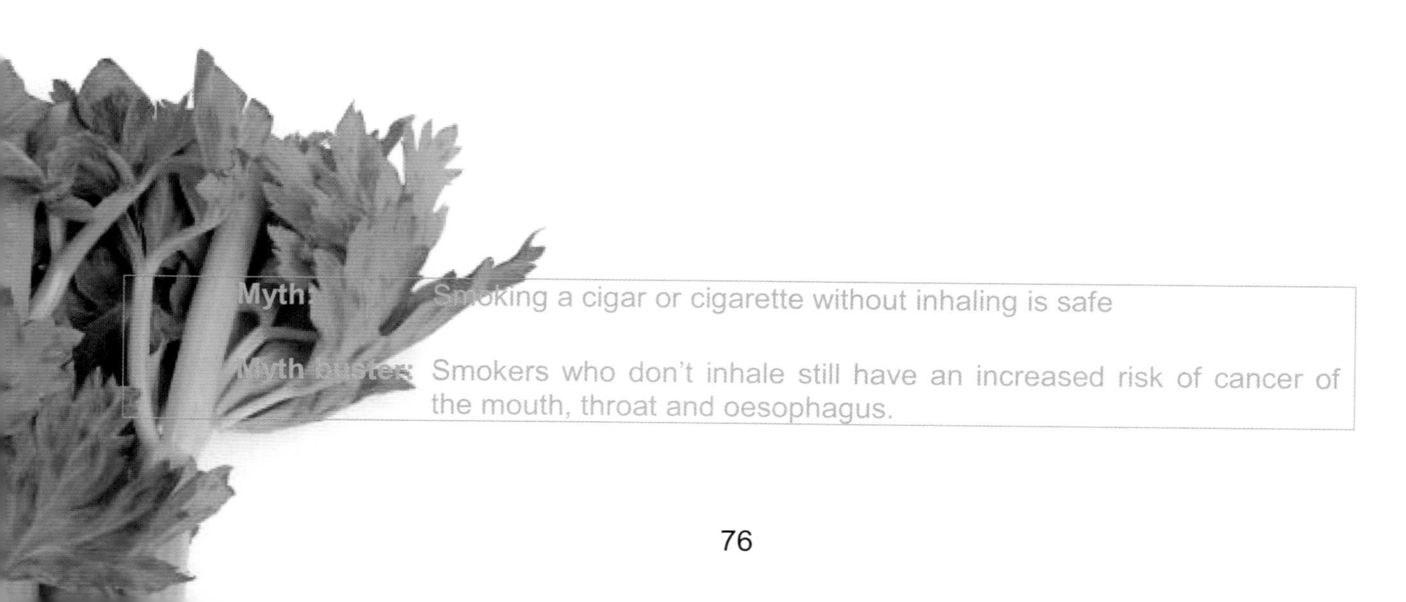

Myth: Smoking a cigar or cigarette without inhaling is safe

Myth buster: Smokers who don't inhale still have an increased risk of cancer of the mouth, throat and oesophagus.

What resources are available to help?

The statistics show that those who try to stop smoking by themselves have a lower permanent quit rate. For this reason, it is important that you use the help that is on offer. You have several options available. Choose one that suits you, but do make sure that you use one of them. You can use a combination of a few different things if that is right for you.

Your options include attending a Smoking Cessation Clinic (all GP surgeries should now offer smoking cessation advice and/or specially dedicated Smoking Cessation Clinics), or using a Quit Smoking Programme.

Clinics can usually offer a variety of support to suit you, from individual to group sessions. They will sometimes offer evening appointments if you have trouble getting away from work.

Stop smoking clinics will give you up to date advice regarding the best way for you to stop and will design a plan for you to follow. They will make an assessment of which aids you need to help you in your attempt. These include Nicotine Replacement products and medication such as Buproprion or Varenicline which help reduce the cravings as you withdraw from nicotine.

If you feel that you do not want to attend a clinic, many good chemists now offer Quit Smoking Programmes and there are now some web sites available for stop smoking support. Take a look on: www.gosmokefree.co.uk and www.newash.org.uk

These programmes take you through all stages of the process from psychologically preparing yourself to maintaining your quit rate long term. There are also Smoking Quit lines available for telephone support and advice using trained counsellors:

NHS Smoking Helpline: 0800 169 0 169

QUITLINE: 0800 00 22 00

Beth's top tip:
Instead of carrot or celery sticks, why not try a cinnamon stick. Not only can you chew on it but you can also inhale through it to make a great natural inhalator

"There are admirable potentialities in every human being. Believe in your strength and your youth. Learn to repeat endlessly to yourself, "It all depends on me"

Andre Gide

What is Nicotine Replacement Therapy?

Nicotine is one of the ingredients in cigarette smoke. It is a very highly addictive substance and as such is responsible for the need to smoke, once hooked. When addicted to nicotine, if you don't get it, your body craves it, making it difficult to give up smoking.

The idea behind Nicotine Replacement Therapy (NRT) is that if you use it during your attempt to quit smoking, it replaces the nicotine from the cigarette and therefore reduces your cravings, which are the main reason most people find it hard to quit.

Research shows that people who use NRT during an attempt to quit are more likely to succeed.

NRT should be started as you start your attempt to quit and continued for several weeks until the worst cravings pass. This is usually over a period of 8-12 weeks.

NRT can be used during pregnancy.

You should use NRT in reducing doses over this period of time, weaning yourself off it, to stop. Nicotine is addictive in any form, including NRT, so you should not continue to use this long term. NRT is available in several different forms such as patches, micro-tabs, lozenges, inhalators, nasal spray and gum. It is available to buy over the counter and also on prescription from your GP.

Have a look at the "Fagerström test" in your Personal Health Plan on page 142, to determine how dependent you are on nicotine. From here you can work out the strength of the product you are likely to need.

As a rough guide, if you have a low dependency, you may only need the lowest strength NRT, if you have a medium dependency, you will need the medium strength product and high dependency, the higher strength. There may however be some overlap in this and flexibility may be needed in what strength you use.

You can also download information regarding the current Nicotine Replacement guidelines from the National Institute for Clinical Excellence

www.nice.org.uk/page.aspx?o=30631

A patient copy of this guidance can be obtained from the NHS Response Line on:

telephone: 0870 1555 455
by quoting the ref: N0084

What if I get addicted to Nicotine Replacement Therapy?

If you use NRT in a reducing dose, over a period of several weeks only, this should not be a problem.

Occasionally people do continue to use NRT beyond the recommended time. This is not advisable. Nicotine in any form does have the effect of raising your blood pressure and can cause an increase in headaches, sleep disturbance and anxiety. However it is still much less dangerous than cigarette smoking itself.

"Nicotine patches are great. Stick one over each eye and you can't find your cigarettes"

Author unknown

What about Buproprion Hydrochloride?

This is a medicine that can be used to help you quit smoking. It is thought to work on the brain's addictive centres and works by reducing cravings. This product is only available on prescription.

It should be started a week or two before your quit deadline as the drug takes this amount of time to reach its optimal effect. You start on a low dose for the first week and then increase to a higher dose and should continue for 6-8 weeks.

Buproprion has been shown to increase your chances of success in quitting.

It cannot be taken if you have epilepsy, an eating disorder or are pregnant or breast feeding.

Have you heard of Varenicline?

This is the newest drug that is available for help in quitting smoking. It works by blocking the sites on the nerves at which nicotine normally attaches. This has the effect of stopping the pleasurable feelings of smoking and also of reducing the cravings associated with nicotine withdrawal.

Early work with this drug is extremely positive and success rates are high, but as the medicine still has very little long term safety testing, as it is so new on the market, doctors are being advised not to use this as a first line treatment as yet. Your doctor may want to prescribe it however, if you have been unsuccessful in previous attempts, using other products.

As with Buproprion, you start Varenicline a week or two before your quit date and can continue it for 8-12 weeks.

Alternative therapies?

There are those who are certain that alternative therapies have helped them. At this point medical research is undecided as to whether they are effective but the therapies that would appear to be most promising are hypnosis and acupuncture. If you are to go this route, please make sure that you find a registered practitioner. Here are some organisations that you could contact:

British Complementary Medicine Association.
PO Box 5122
Bournemouth BH8 OWG

telephone: 0845 345 5977
website: www.bcma.co.uk

Institute of Complementary Medicine

telephone: 020 7237 5165
website: www.icmedicine.co.uk

Sally's story

Sally is 40 years old and works full time in an office. She has smoked 15 cigarettes a day since she was 16 years old. She has had a chest infection for the previous 3 winters and came back to see her GP again last winter, with another. She had tried to give up smoking after her last chest infection and went "cold turkey" following a week of being unwell and smoking virtually nothing over that week. She was successful for a month but started again when her son got into trouble at school. She felt really angry with herself for "failing" and found that because she was stressed and angry with herself, she actually went back to smoking more.

She felt happy to set a dead-line for her quit attempt, as she had no trouble doing this last time, but needed some strategies put in place to help with this attempt, to prevent relapse as happened before.

She attended a Quit Smoking Clinic and was given advice and Nicotine Replacement Patches to help with the cravings which she had found difficult last time. We looked at ways of preventing relapses in times of stress, as happened previously. She found a relaxation exercise helpful and got really good at using it for stress relief in all sorts of different situations, including at work. We talked about the importance of "Time Out" or "me focused time," in dealing with stress and looked at ways of managing her week so that she was able to fit this in. She works full time and has 2 teenage children, but managed a twice weekly Pilates class. She fitted this in by co-ordinating one class a week, when one of her sons was at the sports hall doing football training. The other class she managed when she went straight from work. Her boys had a short time alone at home before her husband got back from work. She found the class especially good for de-stressing before she went home and found that she was much calmer in dealing with her boys as a result.

She found the cravings not nearly as bad when she had the Nicotine Replacement Patches but still put on 3kg (7lb) over the first couple of months, because she was picking more, especially in the evenings or at the weekend, when her mind was less active. She recognised this and kept a supply of carrot or celery sticks in the fridge that she could keep her hands busy with. She stopped putting on weight as a result but couldn't lose the extra pounds.

Sally met a friend in her Pilates class, who had given up smoking the previous year, and they decided that they would start swimming together once a week at their local pool to help with losing weight. The only way of fitting this into her week was to get up early and go before work. This meant that her boys would have to walk to school that morning rather than being dropped in the car on her way to work. Sally surprised herself at how well she was able to keep this up and found that having the incentive of meeting her friend at the pool, and not wanting to let her down, was enough to get her up early. After getting used to the early morning, she found that she really enjoyed feeling that she had done something constructive, while most people were still lying in bed. After building up her stamina to be able to swim continuously for half an hour, she found that she lost 5 out of the 7lb she had put on. She felt great and better toned than she had for years and she and her husband are looking forward to a weekend away next month, paid for with the money that she saved in a jar when she stopped smoking.

Sally has not had a chest infection yet this winter.

My thoughts

Sally is in a strong position at the outset of her attempt to quit smoking. She has had repeated chest infections which are a direct result of her smoking habit and she is fully aware of this. The need to stop comes from within. Her motivation to stop is therefore high. Research has shown that, the more highly motivated a person is, the more likely they are to be successful in their attempt.

It might surprise you to know however that, figures show that 80% of smokers try and quit alone, but 95% of these go back to smoking. Using all help available to you for your attempt will improve your success.

Use the quit lines, web sites and clinics. Take up the offer of nicotine replacement therapy. Get your friends and family on board. Sally was far more successful when she did.

Psyching yourself up for and getting through, the initial attempt is of huge importance however, maintaining your smoke free habit is of equal weight.

Pre-planning your quit attempt will possibly make the difference between you being successful or not. If you recognise possible pitfalls before they arise and put in place a safety net, you can be prepared.

Sally recognises that stress is a trigger and uses a relaxation exercise and a Pilates class to help her with this. Exercise is doubly beneficial, as it is a great tension buster and also helps keep your weight down. Pilates is not aerobic enough to help with weight loss, but is great for improving your muscle tone and is a really good, almost meditative form of exercise. Sally found that swimming was a better way to lose weight. This is because it is a more aerobic form of exercise and therefore better at burning calories.

Sally had previously attempted stopping smoking. Of note, was how hard she took it when she slipped. Be kind to yourself, if like her, you do. Of course it's important to be focused and stay on track, but if you waver, think of this as a minor deviation off course. Remember, this is about a life time of change. In the grand scheme, this slip will mean nothing, as long as you see it that way. Pick yourself up. Start again. Think about where you went wrong. Write it down and plan what you will do next time if the situation recurs.

Smoking
(Get your butt out of here)

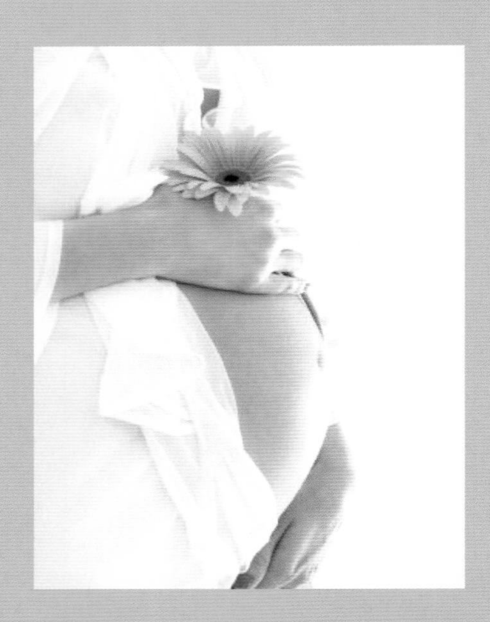

Remember

- Smoking is the biggest cause of ill health in the UK
- Passive smoking can damage your health
- Smoking in pregnancy may damage your baby
- If you smoke near your children, you could damage their health
- The most successful way to quit is to set a deadline and stop completely
- No matter how old you are, quitting smoking has immediate and long lasting health benefits
- Use all the resources available to help you if you want to quit

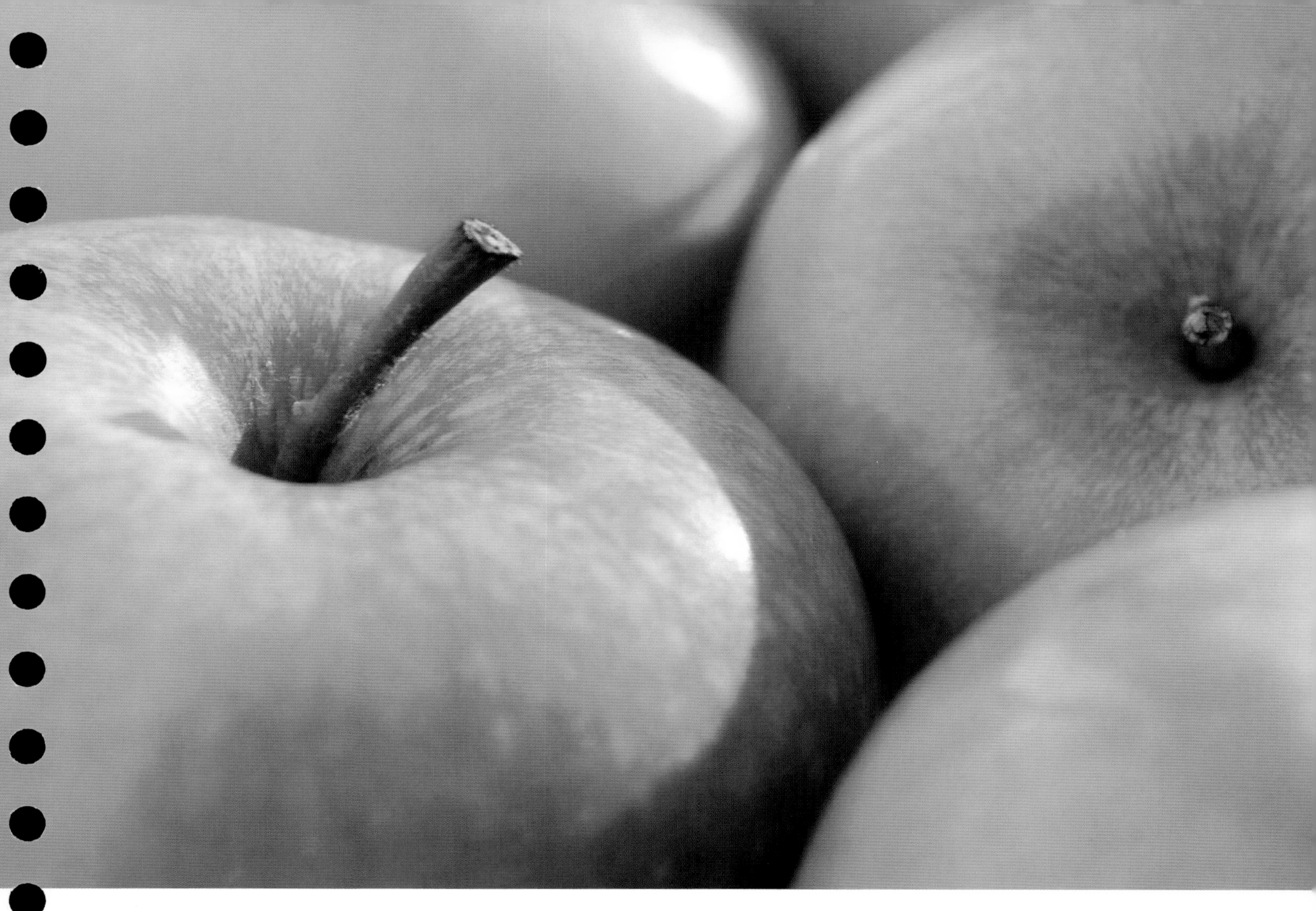

Congratulations

You now have the foundations of what you need to know, in order to lead a healthy life.

I have taken you through weight, diet, exercise, alcohol and smoking. You can see that the basics are actually very simple. Good health is not rocket science. It is feeling great and being able to achieve the most out of life, because you are working with your body and not against it.

Put those changes into action and you will never look back. You will look and feel better than you have ever done. Your enjoyment of life will multiply.

When you feel good about yourself, you will find many things fall into place. You will feel fitter and sexier. Your confidence will grow. As a result, the way you interact with people will blossom and your relationships with your partner, children, friends and work colleagues will improve.

Feeling physically and emotionally stronger you will find that you are keen to tackle all sorts of things that you never thought were possible. Your life will become richer and more fulfilled as a result.

Take a look at the next section on "Make a permanent healthy lifestyle change" and I will show you how to do it.

Good health is just around the corner

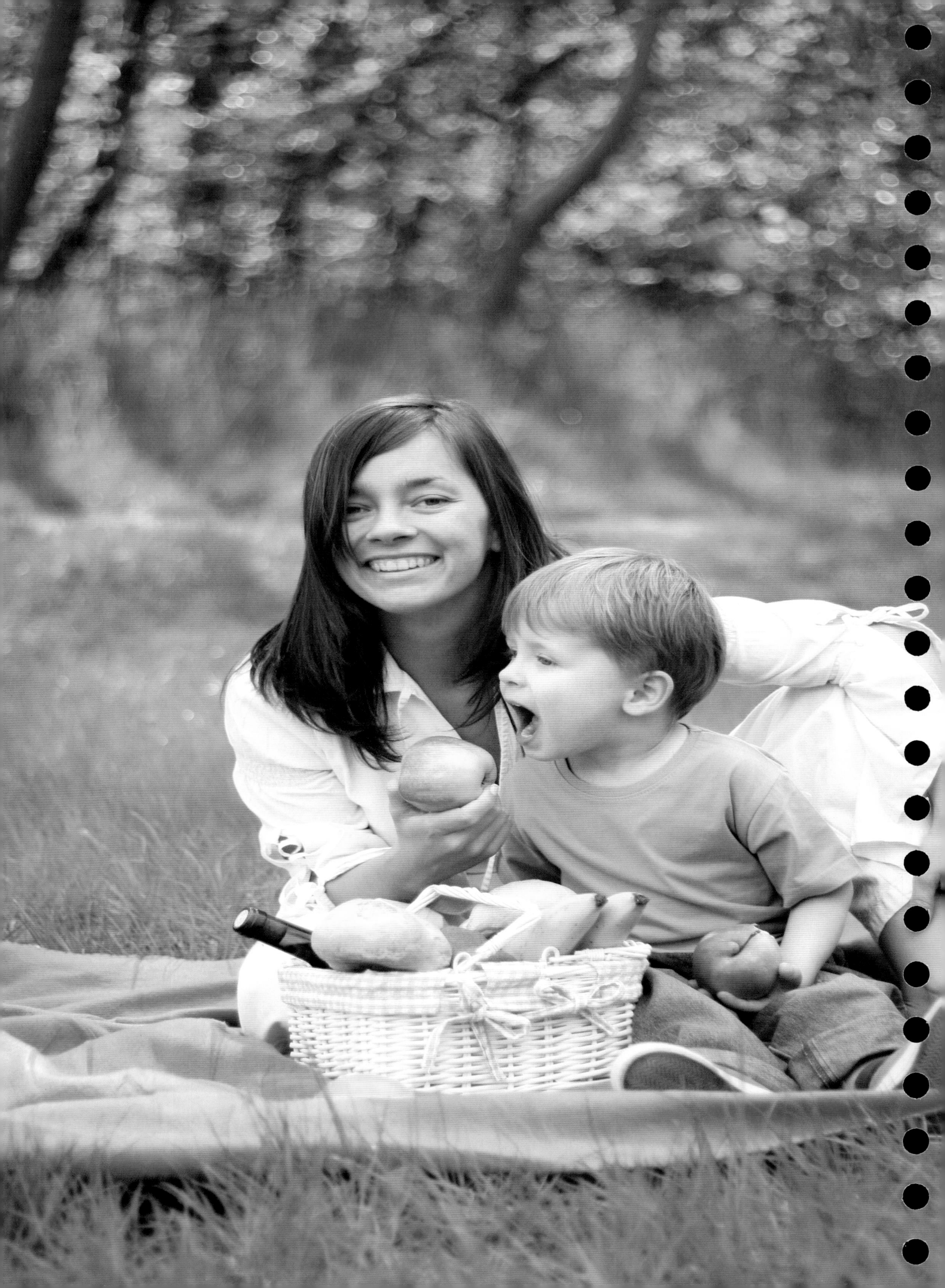

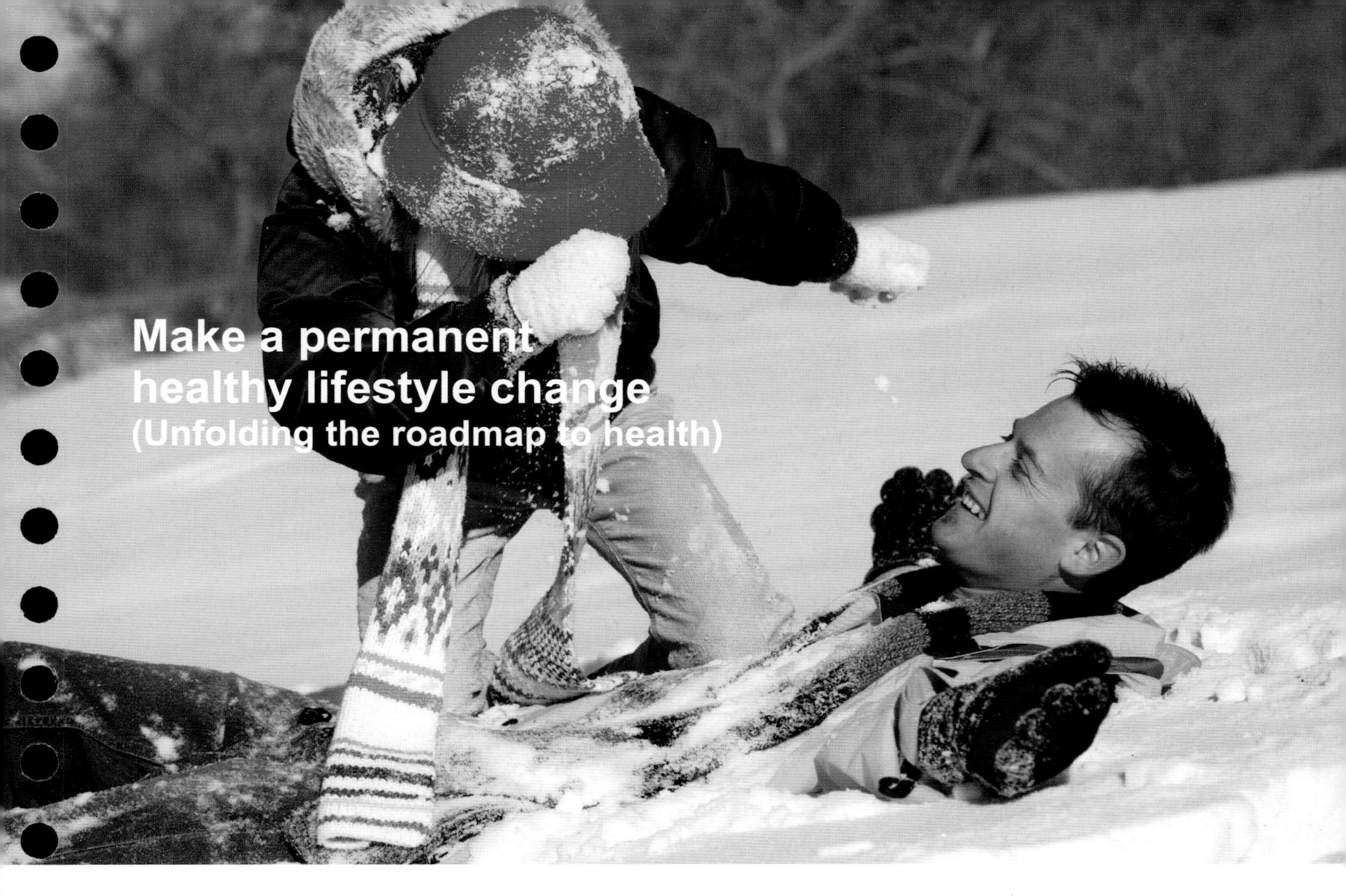

Make a permanent healthy lifestyle change
(Unfolding the roadmap to health)

Now with a good grasp of what you need to know, you are ready to look at how to incorporate those changes into your life.

How can we put all this into action? You have the knowledge base; I will show you how you can use it.

No matter whom you are, or what your circumstances, a healthy lifestyle is achievable. This section on "Make a permanent healthy lifestyle change" will give you the tools that you need to convert your knowledge into action. You will see what you are capable of. It is not about changing the world overnight. It is about taking steady, small steps. Building gradually upon what you already know, tackling things that you feel comfortable with and challenging yourself when you feel ready.

I will show you how with vision and positive language you can motivate yourself. I will teach you how to tackle change effortlessly. I will demonstrate how to set yourself goals that you can attain and I will give you the techniques to enable you to build these things into your life in a sustainable fashion.

I will show you how you can make the very best of what you have. Your potential is huge.

The change that you seek is within you

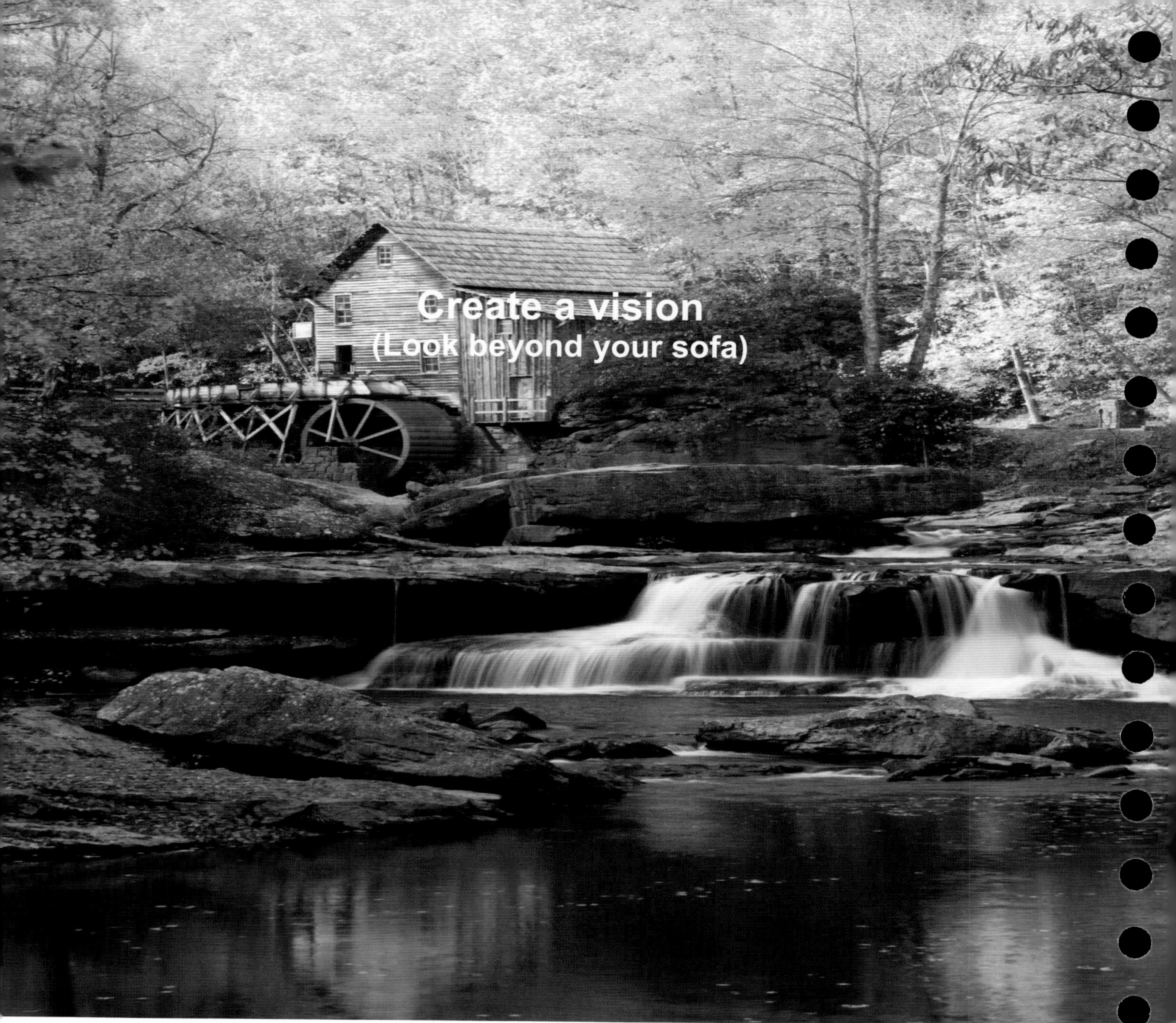

Create a vision
(Look beyond your sofa)

What is a vision and what is its purpose?

When planning anything, it is helpful to know what you want to achieve before you start. Most of us wouldn't set off on a journey, without knowing where we were headed. Your goal is your end point, your final destination. Your vision is one of the tools that you can use to get you there. It is the fuel in your car or the energy in your legs. It is a positive image that you create for yourself in your mind to give you the boost and emotional energy that you need. You can have one or many to help you on your way.

The idea is that you repeatedly refer to your vision in your mind. You can keep it in your head, which means that you can keep going back to it, wherever you are and whatever your circumstances. This is particularly useful, if you find yourself wavering at a weak moment, to prevent you falling off the wagon. Alternatively you can write it down. Keep it with you in your wallet or in your Personal Health Plan, to remind yourself of your dream. The more you do, the more likely it will become a reality.

How do I find my vision?

Spend a few minutes in a quiet room. Close your eyes. Picture in your mind what it is that you want to achieve. Don't think about what you don't want. Think about what you do want.

Here are some ideas:

It might be walking into a room full of smokers and being offered a cigarette and refusing calmly, yet assertively. It might be saying to someone who asks, "no I don't smoke…I gave up a year ago."

It could be you meeting some people you haven't seen for a while. You walk into a room feeling great and they look at you with new eyes and say, "Hey, you look fantastic."

You are walking to the end of the road, without getting short of breath. You are crossing the line at the end of a race, or reaching the top of a hill on your bicycle that you thought you would never be able to get up.

Imagine waking up on a Sunday morning without a hangover, feeling fresh and ready to start the day with vigour.

Now imagine how it would feel to have achieved; how good it is? Store that memory. Tap into it regularly. You can use this vision several times a day if you want.

Your vision may change as you achieve your goals and move on, but always try and keep with you a positive image that you can dip into at will.

What is the difference between a vision and a goal?

There is some overlap here, but essentially your vision is a positive snapshot along the path to your goal. Your goal is your end point. Your vision is an emotional boost that you can use to propel you towards your goal.

For instance, using the example above of the vision being that your friends see you with new eyes looking and feeling great, the goal attached to this might be to eat healthily and to exercise 5 times a week from now on.

"I was always looking outside myself for strength and confidence, but it comes from within. It is there all the time"

Anna Freud

How can deep relaxation help me?

Deep relaxation can be a really effective stress reliever as well as a powerful aid to you visualising and achieving your goals.

When you are in a state of deep relaxation, your subconscious mind is far more open to suggestion. If you use some time when you are in deep relaxation to think about your vision; to feel how good it would feel to achieve it, not only does it become easier for you to tap into at other times, but it makes it more concrete; more real.

I will show you a deep relaxation exercise on page 90. You can do this anywhere that you can find a quiet spot in which you won't be disturbed. I do it both at home and in my office at work sometimes. You can even do it in a quiet place outside. It takes about 10 minutes. The more you do it, the better you get at it, and after a few times you can very quickly, take yourself into really deep relaxation.

The first time you do the exercise, it is helpful if someone reads the narrative to you in a gentle, slow, calm voice. Once you get the sequence into your head, you will be able to do it without help. If you don't have anyone to read it to you or if you find it difficult to memorise, you could tape yourself talking and make your own deep relaxation tape.

Before you start, think of what you would like to focus on when you are deeply relaxed. For the purpose of this exercise, I will use calmness, relaxation and confidence but you can use anything you want. This might be one or two of your ideas on your health plan. Make it a positive focus. For example you could picture yourself at the end of the first week of giving up smoking. Imagine how proud and how much better in yourself you would feel; how good your food would taste and how much your sense of smell would be improved. You could think about how confident you would feel for having lost some weight, or how well you will feel coming into work, without a hangover. Use all your senses. Try and make your vision as real as possible.

Make sure you visualise positive images

Negative thoughts can be really easy to store and seem to jump to the front of our minds when we have a low moment. Sometimes they dominate thoughts without us even recognising what they are. This can be especially so, if you have poor self esteem or are being constantly told by someone close to you that you are no good or worthless.

Recognise these. Their only purpose is to bring you down. Once you recognise them, they will be easier to deal with.

You are in control of them. If you can visualise a negative image, you can see a positive one just as easily. If you find yourself drifting off into negative thoughts, make a conscious effort to say, "I will not let this take over." Force yourself to block it, even if it keeps coming back. The more you do it, the easier it will get. Replace the negative thought with a positive one. This might be your positive vision or even a positive mantra such as:
"I know I can do it."

Set the scene for deep relaxation

Sit comfortably. Take the phone off the hook. Sit upright with your legs uncrossed and with your arms resting lightly on your upper thighs. Close your eyes.

The first stage, progressive relaxation, is designed to relax all the muscles in your body. It is helpful if you have thought of a colour that you find particularly calming before you start the exercise so that if you have someone reading you the deep relaxation sequence described on page 90, they already know what colour to tell you to visualise.

Think of a scene which for you epitomises calm. The most relaxing thing you can think of. If someone is reading the sequence to you, tell them about it in as much detail as you can, so that they can describe it to you, during the exercise. Make sure that you use as many of the senses of sight, touch, taste, sound and smell to make the scene as realistic as possible.

For me, I imagine lying in a rowing boat on a calm lake, which is surrounded by mountains. The warm early morning sun is on my face and there is no-one else on the lake. Every time the oar dips into the water, I see the ripples spreading over the otherwise glassy surface and I tell myself that for every oar stroke I will become more deeply relaxed.

Everyone's idea of calm is different. Choose the picture in your head which best suits you. It might be water, the beach, or mountains. Choose your own.

Once you have completed the progressive relaxation stage, spend a couple of minutes visualising your scene of calmness.

Having done this, you will be very deeply relaxed. You can now spend a couple of minutes focusing on what it is that you want to achieve. You may only need a couple of minutes to let an idea or vision, really take shape. Take as long as you need. Your vision will be entirely individual to you. Make it something that will help lead you to your health goal.

When you are ready, you can finish.

Take a look at the next page, you should now be ready to try the deep relaxation exercise.

"We all have ability. The difference is how we use it"

Stevie Wonder

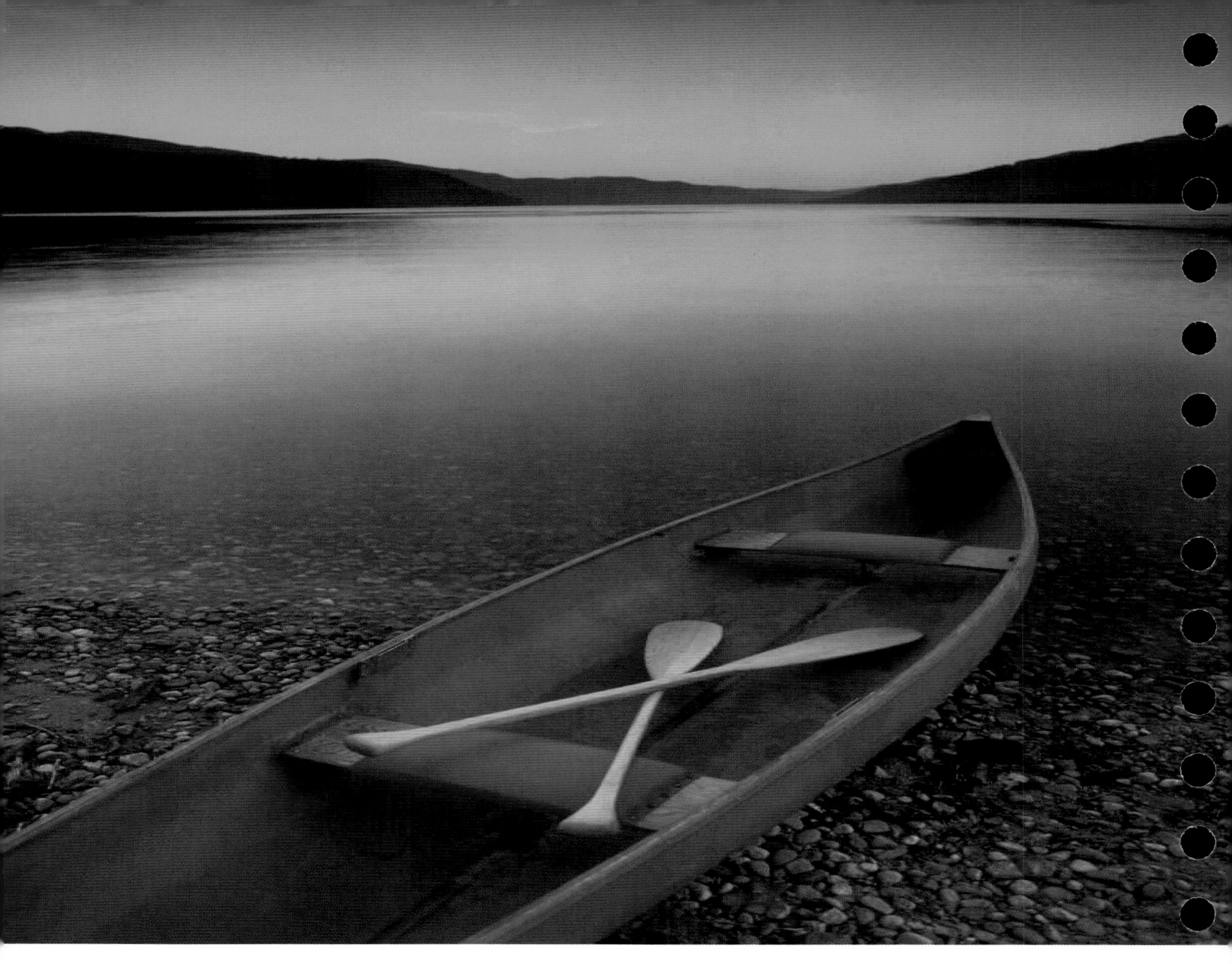

The deep relaxation exercise

Close your eyes. Concentrate on your breathing. I want you to take slow deep comfortable breaths in and out. Focus on the sensation that when you take a deep breath in, that the air is cool and that when you breathe out that your breath is warm. Keep breathing slowly in and out, keeping your mind on the coolness on the breath in, and the warmth on the breath out.

I want you to imagine your eyelids feeling really heavy and relaxed. Really heavy and relaxed. Allow that feeling of relaxation to spread up over the muscles of your forehead, to the top of your head, then the back of your head and spreading down to the back of your neck. The muscles in your face and jaw are relaxing and your head and neck are now feeling really comfortable.

That lovely feeling of relaxation is spreading across your shoulders and down through your upper arms. It is moving to your lower arms and your hands and you can feel all the tension in your upper body flowing away through the tips of your fingers. Feel the tension flowing away through the tips of your fingers.

You are starting to feel really relaxed now and that wonderful calm in your upper body is moving down from your neck and shoulders, down your spine, into your lower back, your buttocks and your thighs. Feel the muscles in your lower legs and feet relax and the last bit of tension in your body flowing away from the tips of your toes.

Your whole body is now feeling beautifully relaxed.

Imagine above your head there is a ball of (your colour) light. It's calm and peaceful and starts to stream down over you and soon your whole body is bathed in the light.

Mentally scan your body to see if there are any remaining areas of tension. Take your mind to that area and focus your thoughts there.

Give the tension a shape. Imagine what it looks like and what it feels like to touch. Does it have a texture or smell? Now imagine it is filling with light and becomes so flooded with it that the shape cannot keep its original form. Your body is swathed in warmth and light. You are feeling more relaxed than you have ever felt before.

Now picture in your mind, your scene of relaxation (describe the scene). Spend a couple of minutes enjoying it. With each moment you spend in it you will become more deeply relaxed.

Take your mind to what it is that you want to focus on. Spend a couple of minutes enjoying your positive thoughts (if you have someone reading this to you, they should give you a couple of minutes of quiet to focus your mind).

Because you are so deeply relaxed, when you are finished with this exercise, you will continue to feel so. You will carry away with you a feeling of calmness, relaxation and confidence. It won't matter where you are or what you are doing, but you will feel a deep inner calm, relaxation and confidence. Calm, relaxation and confidence.

When you are ready, you can open your eyes, getting used to the light in the room.

"I think a hero is an ordinary individual who finds strength to persevere and endure in spite of overwhelming obstacles. Life shrinks or expands in proportion to one's courage"

Anais Nin

Create a vision
(Look beyond your sofa)

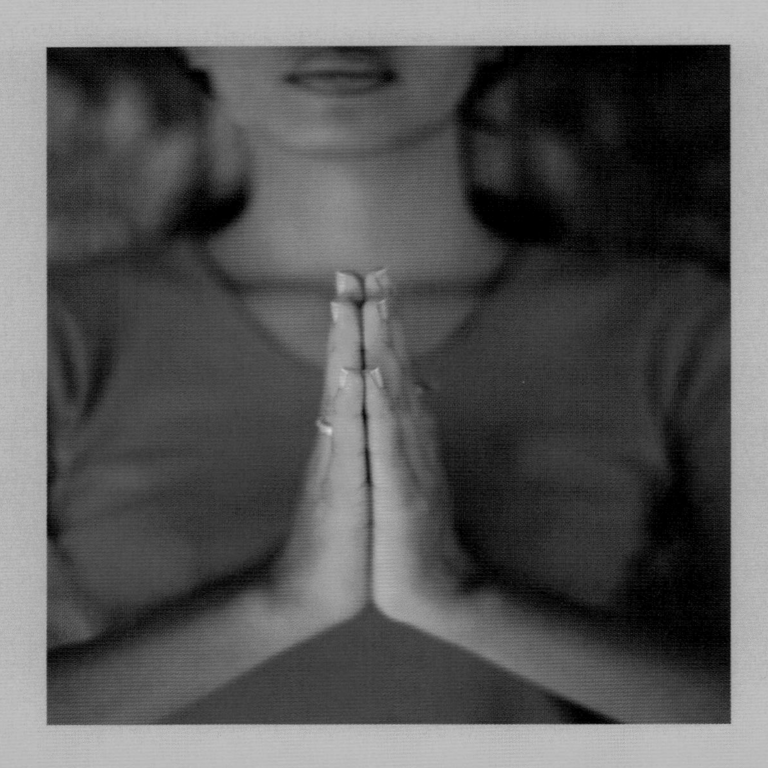

Remember

- Visualize what you want
- Imagine how it would feel to achieve your dream
- Use deep relaxation to reinforce your vision
- Block negative thoughts and images

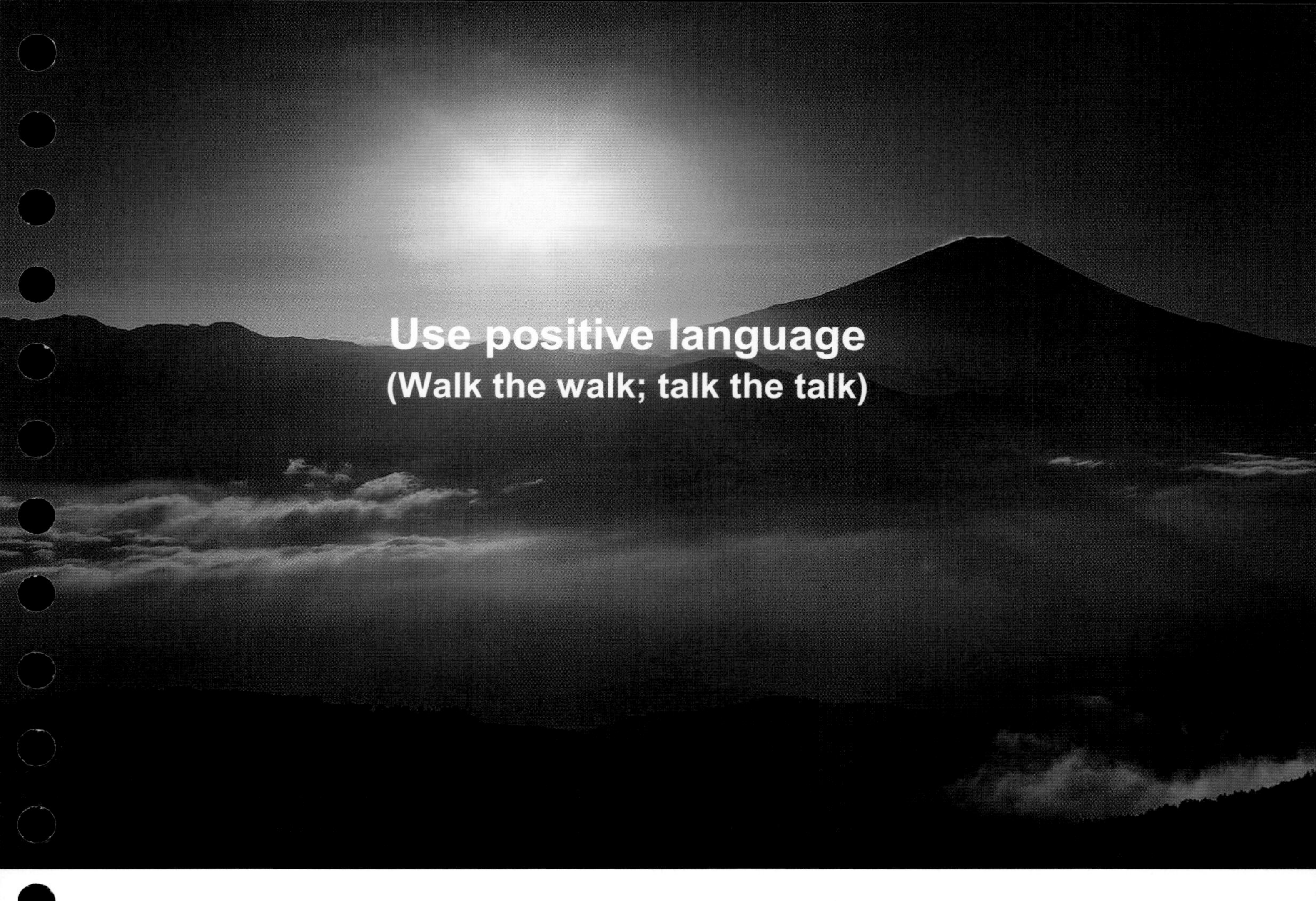

Use positive language
(Walk the walk; talk the talk)

How does positive language make a difference?

Our brains work on two main levels. The conscious and the subconscious. Our conscious brain is that part which is capable of reasoning, questioning and critical thinking. The subconscious brain is working alongside the conscious brain all the time. It soaks up background information and can dramatically change the way in which we see things. Body language is a really good example of this. We are sometimes able to tell far more from this, than what is being said in the spoken word.

What you tell your brain at some level goes in. If it hears a positive message and encouragement, it lifts us. If however it hears that it can't achieve, or that it's no good, it will believe it. Here is a really simple exercise for you to try with someone else, to illustrate this point.

Get your partner to stand with their arm outstretched, parallel to the floor. It is your job to push their arm down, and their job to resist you. Try this first with your partner saying out loud repeatedly, "I'm weak and I'm bad, I'm weak and I'm bad."
Try this next with your partner saying out loud repeatedly, "I'm good and I'm strong, I'm good and I'm strong."

Do you see the difference? When using positive language your partner is far more easily able to resist you.

I saw this done at a conference once and found the difference in the power to resist when being positive, extraordinary. Immediately following the conference I went for a long bike ride on Dartmoor in torrential rain. When getting tired I found myself repeating "I'm good and I'm strong." Instead of coming home fed up and wet, I powered home drenched yet having really enjoyed the ride.

Your subconscious mind can make a huge difference when you are tackling a task. If your attempt at any task is sabotaged by either yourself or someone else saying that it can't be done, your task is much harder.

Keep telling yourself that you can do it. At a subconscious level, in the same way a negative message can bring you down, the positive message will lift you. Avoid using the word "try" as this introduces an element of doubt.

Some examples might be to say:

"I am going to give up smoking" rather than, "I'm going to try to give up smoking."

"I've never done that before but I love a challenge, so count me in," rather than "I can't do that because I've never done anything like that before."

"I am going to do this because I know I can," rather than "I was never any good at that kind of thing, so I don't know if I should."

"I'd love to face that challenge," rather than "I've got no willpower."

It is your job to nurture yourself

When we're of school age, most of us are lucky enough to have people telling us on occasions: "Well done, you did that really well" or "You're really good at that." As an adult, very few of us are in an environment in our relationships or workplace, that praise or congratulate us.

You have to believe you can make changes for yourself.

Even if you don't believe you can, you have to tell yourself repeatedly that you can. At a subconscious level that message will get through and as soon as you start to believe you can do something, the journey becomes easier.

I remember a childhood story about a tiny train which makes the journey to the top of a long steep hill. He is determined to get to the top, despite the fact that a bigger stronger train tells him that he can't. He focuses on one thing: a vision of the top of the hill and he sets off saying: "I think I can, I think I will, I know I can, I know I will" over and over again. This is a great mantra, partly because of the sentiment and partly because of the syntax. This is one I use when I'm climbing a long hill on my bike and in the same way that it carried the little engine, it never fails to help me get to the top of a hill.

Positive language is like an emotional "leg up;" it still requires you to focus and do the work, but it makes the job much easier.

"Motivation is the fire from within. If someone else tries to light that fire under you, chances are it will burn very briefly"

Steven R. Covey

 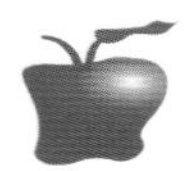

Don't sabotage your own success

Some people fear standing out, because others might think that they're *too* good, or because people might think that they're big headed or arrogant. It is easy to put yourself down, without realising that you are doing it.

You will find that people treat you as you treat yourself. If every time someone compliments you, you say something negative in return, either one of you or both of you will start to believe it. The next time someone gives you a compliment, just say "Thank you."

Enthusiasm for life is infectious. There are some people who light up a room. If you have someone smiling at you and encouraging you, it is hard not to reciprocate. You will find that your positive outlook lifts both you and others too.

Recognise when you are using negative language. If you hear yourself doing it, write down what it was that you said and think of a more positive way that you could say it next time.

For example instead of saying "I'm really bad at getting down to losing weight," you could say "I find losing weight a challenge, but one that I'm *going* to tackle."

Use page 145 in your Personal Health Plan to record your positive thoughts.

Encourage yourself

Most people wouldn't think twice about encouraging their children. Do it to yourself. Face a challenge with "Come on, I'm going to be great" or "I can do anything" and don't forget to congratulate yourself if you've done well.

You don't have to blow your own trumpet but it's really healthy to be quietly confident in one's own ability.

Think of a person who you know, who projects confidence. Most of us know one. You may have thought on occasions, "I wish I could be like that."

You can.

Believe in yourself. You can do it

The point at which you achieve your first goal, will be the moment at which you will know that you *can* succeed. If you have achieved something that you thought was impossible at the start, your self belief will grow. Each subsequent goal will become easier. Not because you are setting yourself easier targets, but because you believe in yourself.

Try this today

Choose one of these things and have a go. Have fun.

- Write down 5 things that you like about yourself
- Think of something you have done in the past that has made you laugh and tell someone about it
- Write down 5 things you like about your partner and give the list to them
- Write down something about yourself that you would like to change and next to that write down how you will go about changing it
- Say something nice to someone you don't normally get on with

Use positive language
(Walk the walk; talk the talk)

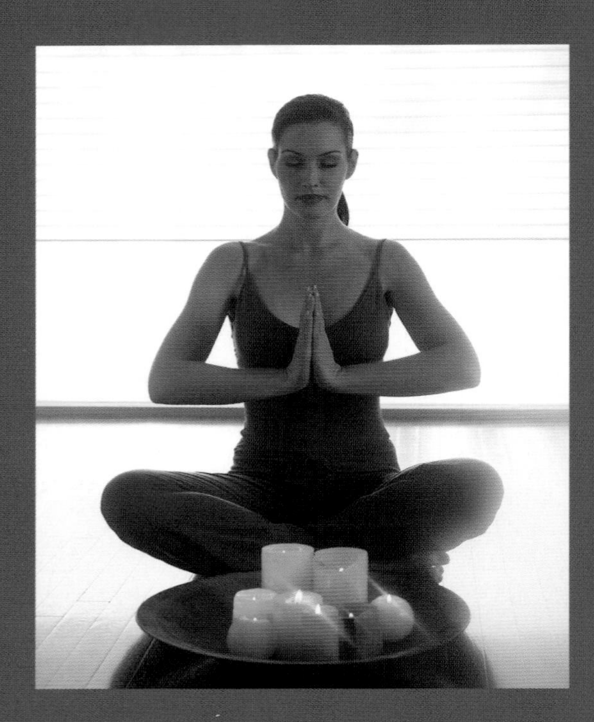

Remember

- Use positive language to focus your mind and to ...make you strong
- Recognise negative language and stop using it
- Tell yourself you can
- Congratulate yourself regularly
- Self belief is infectious. If you believe in yourself, ...others will believe in you too

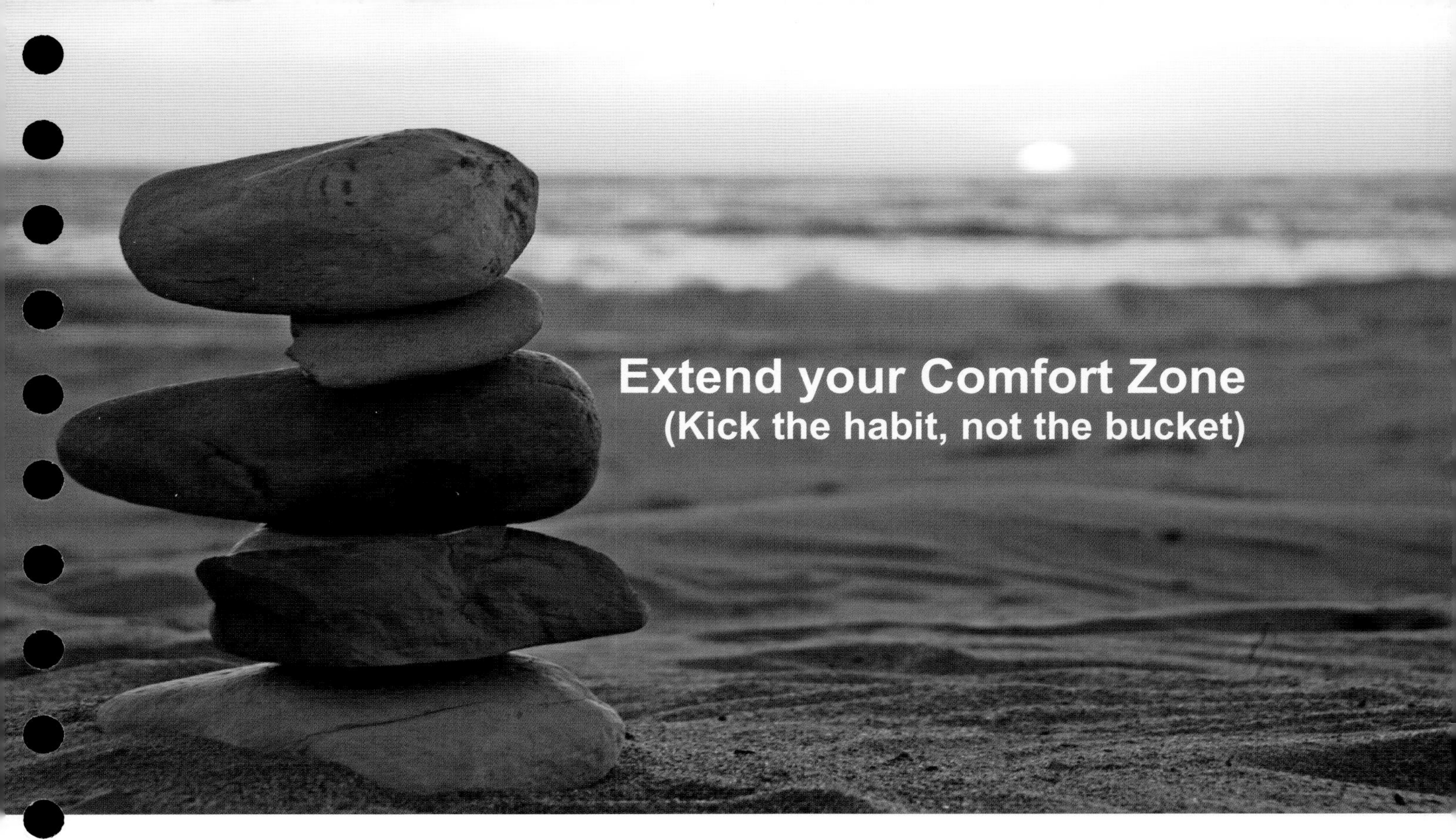

All of us have a Comfort Zone. This is the range of activities within which we operate with ease. Some of us have bigger Comfort Zones than others. They can be of many different types including emotional, social, and physical. Unless we challenge them they will remain as they are or even shrink.

I like to think of Comfort Zones in this type of model:

Panic Zone

⇗

Challenge Zone

⇗

Comfort Zone

The Comfort Zone

Comfort Zones are created by repeating certain behaviours until they become a habit. Once so, we become accustomed to that way of working and incorporate this pattern in our subconscious mind as to what is "normal" for us. This is great if the pattern is a positive one, but sometimes we engage in negative activities or language, which subsequently become our norm and can trap us in our Comfort Zone. An example that I hear frequently is "I've got no willpower." Other excuses not to engage in change include:

"I would do it if I had more time/money"
"I'll change when things are better for me"
"I would if it wasn't for my partner/parents/children

Making excuses by blaming external forces or other people sets you up to fail. The door for any attempt is closed and your Comfort Zone stays as it is.

The Challenge Zone

The Challenge Zone is the area just outside your Comfort Zone. This area is one you don't normally stray into and if you do, you feel challenged but not threatened. The challenge can be really enjoyable. You will become accustomed to repeatedly doing an activity from the Challenge Zone and if done enough, this will become a habit, and so it will be incorporated into your Comfort Zone.

The Panic Zone

The Panic Zone is way outside your area of comfort and can be stressful to enter. Repeatedly going there will decrease your levels of anxiety and may be a more rapid way of stretching your Comfort Zone. Some people thrive on this kind of adrenaline. However others find the experience traumatic. The risk of stretching yourself too quickly is that after one or two attempts you might completely abandon all efforts, so it's generally better to start by tackling your Challenge Zone.

You will find that before long, what was originally in your Panic Zone may be well into your Challenge Zone or even your Comfort Zone.

An example of someone stretching their Comfort Zone too rapidly might be someone who wanted to lose weight, going on a crash diet, rather than opting for slower weight loss. It may take a little longer to get to your target weight by adopting a steady approach; however it avoids failure because of an unmanageable pace and routine.

Why should you extend your Comfort Zone?

If you have a small Comfort Zone, you have fewer things that you feel at ease doing. This means that your life experiences will be less rich. Many of us are guilty of not doing a certain thing, because we feel that it is something that we wouldn't be able to do.

Ask yourself why? You may have a valid reason. But often it is just because you are too under confident, or simply have a mental block or are too ingrained in old bad habits that you decide not to try.

Start the process of change today. Break your routine. Try something different, it can be a really fun and eye opening experience. Simple things to try might be:

- Don't watch TV for 24 hours; engage in a hobby or go for a walk instead
- Get up an hour early and see how much time it opens up in your day
- Sit with a different group of people
- Wear something you wouldn't normally
- Walk to the top of a hill and shout out the first thing that comes into your head as loudly as you can
- Ask someone you don't normally speak to their opinion

Challenging yourself successfully, especially when you present yourself with something that you believed you couldn't do, is extraordinarily satisfying. You will find that your life will become more fun and diverse as a result and your confidence will grow in all sorts of other areas.

Recognise false negative beliefs and challenge them

Sometimes we carry negative behaviours or beliefs around with us from childhood. I left school thinking I was bad at sport because I was someone who didn't enjoy ball sports. I carried that thought around with me for years. Since that time I have taken up swimming and cycling, Kayaking and Tae Kwon-do, none of which were available to me at school, but all of which I now enjoy enormously. It took me years to overcome the sentiment that I was "no good" at sport.

If we recognise these erroneous beliefs for what they are, or even if we don't recognise them as that, but give ourselves the chance to challenge them and therefore change them, we can start to move out of our Comfort Zones.

Recognise the Comfort Zone that you make for yourself and the false beliefs that keep you there; challenge yourself; create a new bigger Comfort Zone and enjoy the confidence it brings you.

Keep at it even if you feel you're not making progress

Of course it can be uncomfortable moving out of your Comfort Zone for the first time. Like anything else, the more you do it, the easier it becomes. If you find that you don't succeed the first time you try, keep going and try again. With each effort you learn something.

I like to use the analogy of children learning to walk. Inevitably they fall repeatedly, before they get the hang of it. Rather than giving up after the first fall they pick themselves up and try again. Not to do so would mean they would never learn to walk.

Enlist the support of those around you

Enlist the help and support of those around you. Get your partner to encourage you to exercise even when you want to give it a miss for a night. Perhaps you can give up smoking with your spouse, get a friend to go along with you to an exercise class or start a healthy lifestyle group at work.

Most GP surgeries now operate Smoking Cessation Clinics. Some offer Lifestyle Clinics. All GPs should have access to counsellors who specialise in alcohol problems. Most GPs will now prescribe medicines to aid weight loss to patients who fulfil certain criteria. There are now some good web sites available to help you with all aspects of giving up smoking, reducing your alcohol intake and losing weight. Use them. You wouldn't walk to the top of a mountain without shoes. Why set yourself a difficult challenge and not use the resources that are there to help? The more support you have from others, the easier your job will be.

Build your foundations well

This is about a lifetime of change. There is no rush. Build your foundations well.

"They always say time changes things, but you actually have to change them yourself"

Andy Warhol

Extend your Comfort Zone
(Kick the habit, not the bucket)

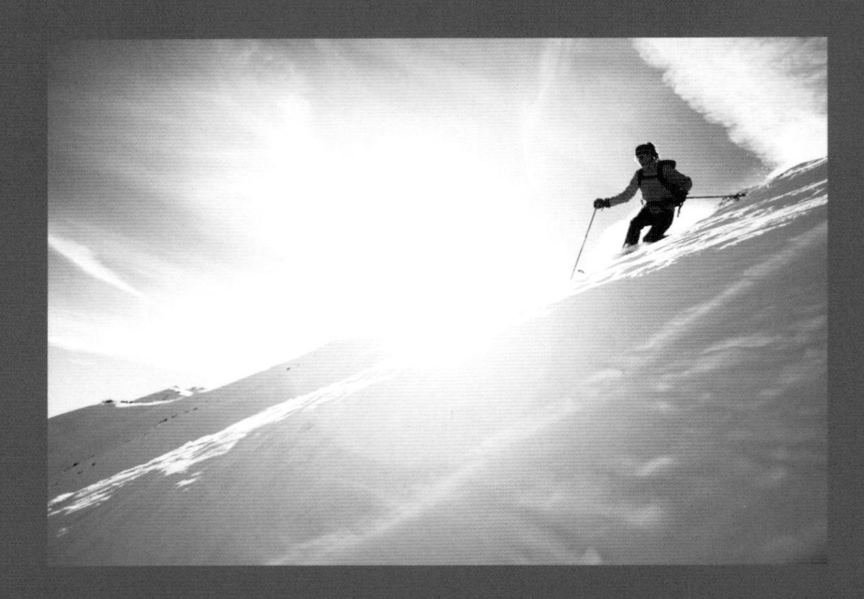

Remember

- Repeating an activity from outside your Comfort Zone gets easier each time you do it
- Recognise negative habits and beliefs that hold you in your Comfort Zone and challenge them
- Push your boundaries gently
- Enlist the support of others
- Use all resources available for help

Set a goal
(How the tortoise beat the hare)

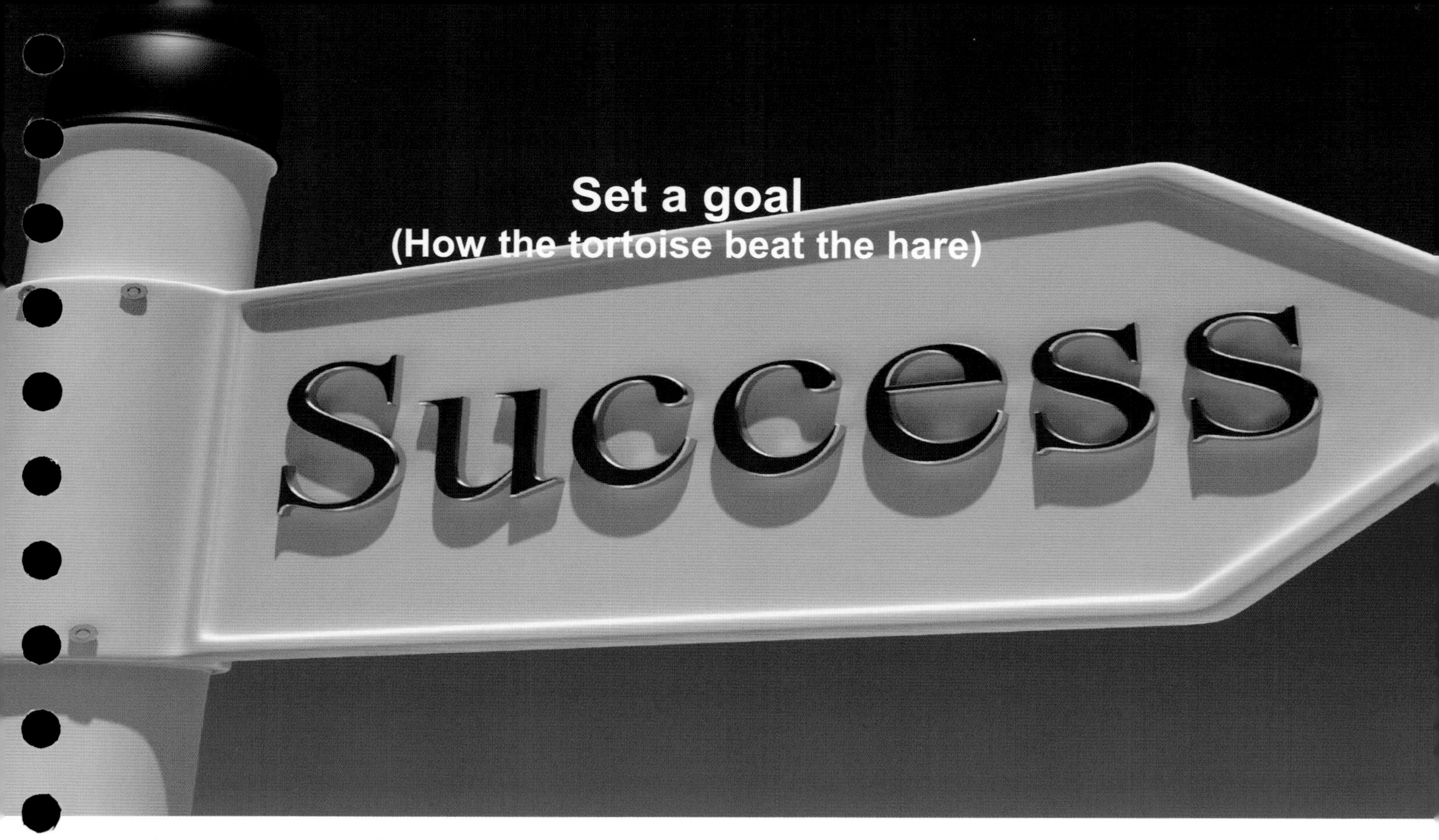

It's very easy to drift through life without knowing where we are going. Life goes by fast. We have one chance at it. All of us are made differently. Some of us thrive on filling every single moment with activities and others prefer space in their lives to simply reflect or just to "be."

Whatever way you choose to live your life, it is important that you get the opportunity to live it in the way that you want to.

With a little planning you are far more likely to be able to do this. It sounds like a contradiction in terms to say that you need to plan to do nothing, but actually sometimes our lives happen around us at such a pace and we seem to have so little control over the flurry of tasks and things to do, that we don't ever get the chance to be still.

Setting a goal gives us the vision of where we want to be. Once we have that aim, then we can set about the task of how to achieve it.

We often focus on what we don't want or don't like about our lives. This challenge is to focus on *what you do want*.

If you find it difficult to see this in your mind, here's a good trick to help:

Imagine that you are walking into the back of a church. It's a funeral. You can see all the people who you love and care about there; your friends and family, your neighbours, people from your work place. One of these people stands up to speak to the congregation about the person's life. When they start, you realise that it's your own funeral. What would you like that person to say about you? How ideally would you like to have lived your life? If your spouse, your children, your best friend and your work colleagues were to speak, how would you like them to describe you?

Take a few quiet moments to think this through and then jot your ideas down in your Personal Health Plan at the back on page 146. This is a good starting point.

The SMART goal

When setting a goal it should fulfil certain criteria. I like to use the acronym SMART to illustrate this. Your goal should incorporate all of the characteristics below.
It should be:

Specific

Measurable

Agreed

Realistic

Time-scaled

Why use a SMART goal?

When you do the "funeral visualisation exercise," you will end up with a piece of paper full of ideals, some of which you do, or have achieved already, some of which you would like to do but haven't got the time/finance/know how, but could do if you had. Some of them however, you know that with the best will in the world you will never achieve. Never say never. What do I mean by this?

Sometimes an idea or a goal seems so huge that despite the desire to achieve, you believe it to be something that you will never do. If you set yourself an enormous task which might seem completely insurmountable for whatever reason, you are setting yourself up to fail. Failure at the first hurdle can be really destructive and can put you off going back and trying again.

Build your foundations slowly

When you start, choose a goal that you feel pretty confident that you can achieve. The physical gain from achieving that goal may not be great, but the emotional gain is huge. This will give you the confidence to tackle another goal, possibly more challenging next time. Bite sized chunks of confidence will grow into a banquet before you know it. Taking lots of small progressive steps, using your last goal as a leg up towards the next and working towards a big end goal, makes the job manageable.

As you achieve more and more you will recognise that you are doing things that you thought you could or would never do. Suddenly the impossible ideals are reality.

The idea of the "SMART" Goal is that if you use this as a framework, you are far more likely to set yourself a goal that you can achieve.

It's helpful to take the SMART goal one step further. Add evaluation and review to your goal tick list. You will find that some goals you will tackle with ease. Look back at what it was that made it so simple to accomplish. You will want to use this for future goal planning. Almost inevitably there will be some tasks that you find far more challenging. It is really important to understand why it was that this was so, especially if you were not successful. Identify what it was that made you stumble and think of an alternative strategy that you can put in place for your next attempt. Make a note of your ideas on your "Goal Evaluation Page" on page 155.

Remember, failure is not making a mistake, but neglecting to use what you have learned to subsequently succeed.

The specific goal

Ideally your goal should be specific. For example rather than saying that you want to cut down on the amount of alcohol that you drink, you should specify by how much. Rather than saying you are going to start walking, you say for example, you're going to start walking for 30 minutes 5 times a week.

This approach immediately frames your goal for you, so you know what you are aiming for.

The measurable goal

This overlaps with the specific goal. The point of this is that you have a barometer of your success. This gives you a sense of achievement when your goal is attained and also allows you to plan further goals from it. For instance if you walk for 30 minutes 3 times a week and cover 1 mile a session for the first year, you might want to increase that to a mile and a half or 2 miles in your second year.

Your goal might be to cut out the packet of crisps that you have every lunch-time with your sandwiches.

The agreed goal

This is all about *you*. The will to tackle a goal must come from *within you*. If you don't have the motivation, the challenge will be far more difficult. For instance it has been shown that the smokers who do best when giving up are those who really want to, not those who have been told that they have to. Pick your own goals. You will be far more likely to succeed if the drive is your own.

The realistic goal

Every goal you set should be a realistic one. It is really easy when filled with enthusiasm when starting a new resolution or fresh project to stretch yourself way beyond your capabilities.

There are a whole load of reasons why big ideas fail. There may be time constraints, physical constraints or how to tackle the idea maybe just too much to get your head around. These hitches may make it difficult to maintain momentum or even can prevent the whole thing getting off the ground in the first place.

If you have big ideas, break your idea down into a series of smaller parts, and then tackle each one as a successive goal. For instance, if you want to cut down on the amount of alcohol that you drink, rather than saying that you are going to give up drinking, you could start with a target of keeping a couple of days a week alcohol free. When you feel comfortable with that, you could look at decreasing the number of drinks that you have on your weekday nights when you do consume alcohol. When you have settled into this routine, you might swap your binge drinking routine on a weekend night, for an amount within your safe limits. At any of these stages you can divert your goal. You might want to add in exercise, healthy eating or quitting smoking into your regime at some point. In this way your goals are progressive and evolve.

The time-scaled goal

Some people are good at working at a steady pace with what is presented to them; some like to put off a task until the last minute while others like to talk about it but just can't to ever seem to get around to the job required of them.

If you put a timescale on your goal, it immediately makes the task a reality. In other words it gives you a dead-line. Make sure that when you give yourself a time-scale that it is a realistic one. If you have set yourself bite sized realistic goals this should be relatively easy to do.

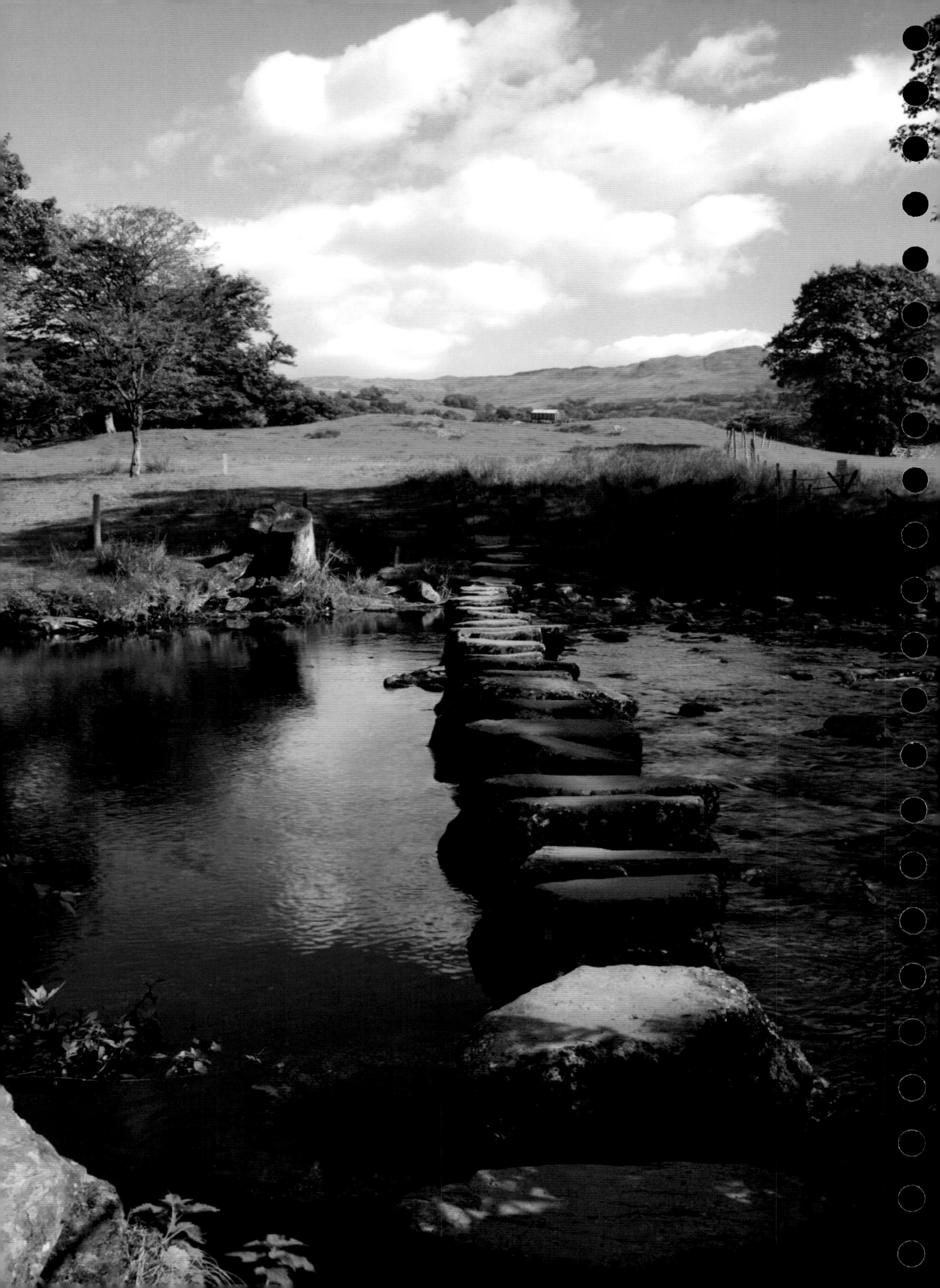

Short, medium and long term goals

When you do the "funeral" exercise, you will find yourself with a whole load of different ideas. Not all of them will be appropriate to tackle, straight away. Some will require you to be at a certain stage in life, for example with children, without children, more financially sound, or retired. Just because you cannot directly embark on them at this moment does not mean that they have to be forgotten. They should become part of your medium or long term plan.

Having an idea of the direction in which you wish your life to go enables you to take control and guide it there. If you lose sight of these things or discount them as being mere dreams, the foundations cannot be laid and they may drift from you.

A good way of identifying what you want your long term goals to be is to spend a few minutes imagining where you would like to be and what you would like to be doing in 10 or 20 years time. If you find this too difficult, think ahead 5 years.

You can use your short term goals to fulfil your medium term goals, which you may in turn use as a stepping stone towards your long term goals.

Of course like everything in life, there needs to be flexibility. Your goals may change as your circumstances or interests change. The important thing is that you are the director of your own life.

Use the page dedicated to your goals in your Personal Health Plan on page 147 to record your short, medium and long term goals.

Balance your goals

A healthy life is a well balanced one. If you direct all your energies into one area of your life, another may suffer.

For instance, to direct all your focus to exercise, to the exclusion of work or family life would in the end be counter-productive and may make your regime unsustainable. If however you balanced your plan by for example involving your family or work colleagues in your exercise regime, you would have better chance of success.

The main areas in most people's lives are:

- Work
- Finances
- Family and friends
- Health, well being and leisure
- Spirituality

Make sure that when you set your goals that you look at all aspects of your life, examining each one individually to ensure that your energies are creating harmony and not disarray.

"The reason that most people never reach their goals is that they don't define them, or ever seriously consider them as believable or achievable. Winners can tell you where they are going, what they plan to do along the way and who will be sharing the adventure with them"

Denis Whatley

Nicki's story

Nicki is 35 and her father had a stroke 6 months ago. He was diagnosed with diabetes several years ago. He ran the local pub and had been overweight for years. Nicki wanted advice as to how she could reduce her risks of becoming diabetic, as in many ways, she had always taken after her father. She was 13kg (2 stone) overweight and her only exercise was the short walk to the bus stop in the morning on her way to work. She worked part time behind the bar at the family pub and drinks were freely available. She smoked, although her smoking habits were quite variable and most of her smoking was done when at work. Since the smoking ban, it had become more difficult to get away and have a cigarette.

There were many areas of Nicki's life that needed focus. We talked about the fact that in order to reduce her risks of diabetes or stroke she would need to do several things which included: stopping smoking, losing weight, exercising more, looking at the kind of foods that she ate and cutting down on the amount of alcohol that she was drinking. As a list this seemed quite overwhelming and Nicki wondered how she would ever go about tackling all of these areas successfully.

We talked about prioritising and goal setting and Nicki came up with a list of what she wanted to achieve over the next 5 years.

Nicki's long term goal: in the next 5 years she will:

- become more healthy, to avoid becoming overweight and having diabetes like her father

Nicki's medium term goal: in the next 12 months she will:

- give up smoking
- lose 1 stone
- have herself and her family eating healthily
- increase her exercise level to 30 minutes 5 times a week
- reduce her alcohol consumption to the recommended level

Nicki's short term goals:

As from next week she will:

- include only healthy snacks for her own and her family's daily packed lunches. She will always take a healthy snack with her rather than buying one at work, to avoid temptation of sweet snacks
- get off the bus a stop early twice a week and walk the remainder of the journey to and from work (she'll need to buy an umbrella for winter!)

In addition, as from next month she will:

- set a date to quit smoking
- increase the number of days that she gets off the bus a stop early to 4 times a week
- have a walk at the weekends with her family

In another 2 months in addition she will:

- keep to the recommended portion sizes of meals
- make a resolution to only use a ready made meal once a week. She will buy herself a teach yourself to cook book, to get some ideas of simple recipes she can use cooking with fresh ingredients
- stay alcohol free on the days that she is not working behind the bar

In addition the following 2 months she will:

- cook fish once a week
- swim 10 lengths at the pool, while her son has his swimming lesson

After a further 2 months in addition she will:

- eat 2 pieces of fruit a day
- swim 20 lengths once a week

The following 2 months she will:

- eat 3 pieces of fruit a day
- swim 30 lengths once a week

In addition after a further 2 months she will:

- use the frying pan only once a week
- swim 40 lengths a week

My thoughts

I have given you an example of what a time-scaled plan might look like over a one year period. Can you see how Nicki has made small changes and gradually built on them? It doesn't matter what order she does them in. The plan needs to suit her needs and should be entirely individual to her. Her arrangement of goals is particularly successful as she has already started her healthy eating and exercise plan, prior to giving up smoking, which will help prevent any weight gain and the exercise sessions will be a really good stress reliever if she is feeling the tension of not having a cigarette. Notice that she is careful not to make too many changes at the time that she sets her deadline for stopping smoking.

You can see that Nicki's plan does not yet fulfil all the requirements of a completely healthy living plan. The idea is to spend time getting used to and enjoying one step, before moving on to the next. Consolidate then build. It doesn't matter if Nicki takes 2-3 years to achieve everything. The important thing is that what she starts, she maintains. If Nicki decides that after a year, she doesn't want to introduce anything new, as long as she continues with the changes already made she will benefit greatly long term; as will her family.

Losing weight is a difficult goal to frame with long term success. What do I mean by this? To specify a certain amount of weight loss is a helpful target but don't be too hung up on this. Far better to set a goal in terms of healthy eating and exercise (which should in turn help you lose weight), than to motivate yourself with kilos or pounds, which could encourage fad or crash diets.

Nick's long term goal is quite general, but both her medium and short term goals feed into her plan and are much more specific.

Set a goal

(How the tortoise beat the hare)

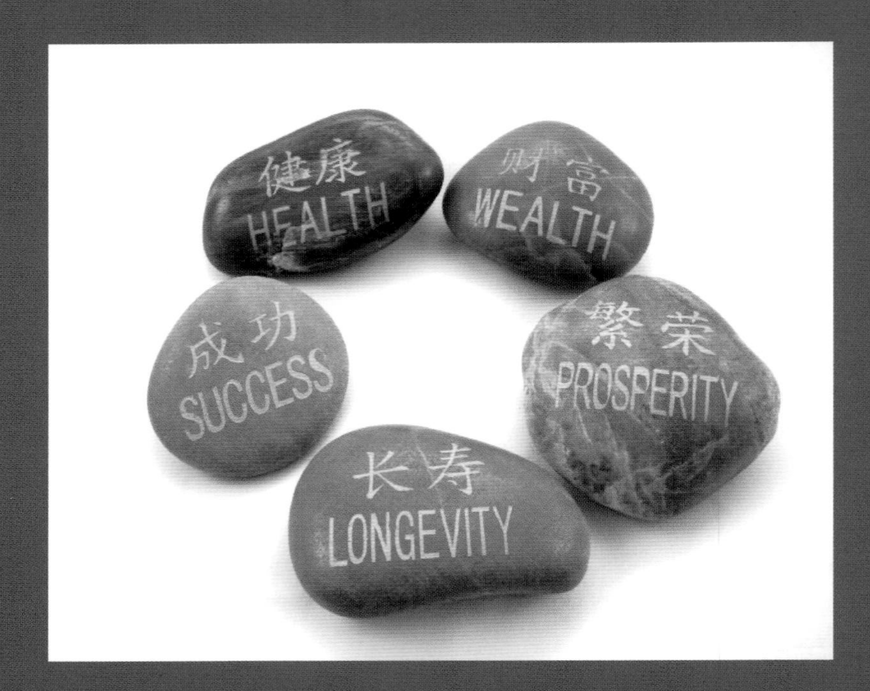

Remember

- Set SMART goals; evaluate and review them
- Keep in mind your long term goals when setting short term ones
- Build your foundations slowly
- Balance your goals

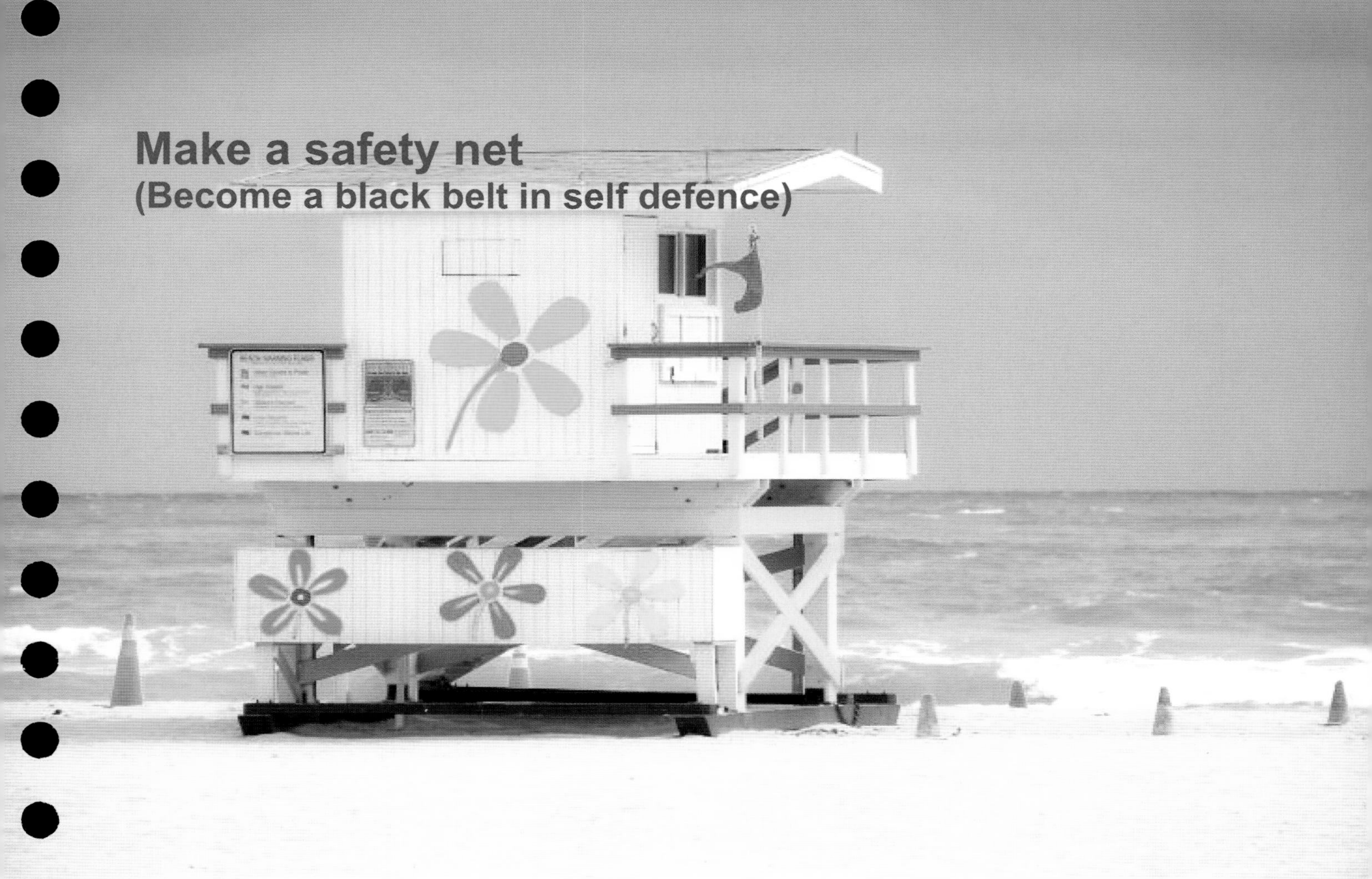

Make a safety net
(Become a black belt in self defence)

The tasks we set ourselves are of varying importance to us. Sometimes if we set ourselves a task which is of extreme importance (weight loss and giving up smoking are right up there at the top of the list for a lot of people), if we “lapse” the effect can be devastating. It can take months for us to regain confidence in ourselves, before we try again and in the meantime it’s not uncommon to rebound into worse habits than before we started.

We need to tackle this in three ways:

1) Start the process by setting realistic goals
2) Acknowledge that you are human
3) Identify obstacles before they occur and put in place strategies to avoid them

1) Set realistic goals

This immediately sets you up to win. Building up a series of smaller successive goals is far easier than tackling one huge one. With each success comes an increase in confidence. Temporary set back over a small goal is not only far easier to overcome, but if you have set about the process by a series of small goals, even if you get only part way through the series, you will have at least tackled and completed part of your overall target. Starting with a huge goal is sometimes so daunting that it doesn’t even get off the ground. If you don’t have smaller bench marks along the way, if you don’t reach your final target, you can feel like you have nothing to show for your efforts. This can be really demoralising.

2) Acknowledge that you are human

What does this mean?

This is all about recognising that with the best will in the world, some of us slip up at times. That's ok. That's part of living a life that is enjoyable and not so stripped of pleasures that we can no longer enjoy it.

Allow yourself treats occasionally. You will have days when you can't be bothered to or just practically can't get out and exercise. You may need more than one attempt at quitting smoking. The important thing is not to be devastated when this happens.

As long as the main thrust of your plan is in the right direction, you are on track. Remember, these are changes that you want to maintain for a life time. If you beat yourself up every time you slip, there will be very little incentive to try again.

It is almost inevitable that we will fall off the wagon periodically. Recognise this. There are plenty of things that you can do to help. In the next few pages I have written about some ways which should guide you with regard to weight, diet, exercise, alcohol and smoking. I call these "safety net" strategies.

Use the "safety net" strategies to visualise what you might do in the eventuality that you did slip. Think of how you might deal with the situation positively to enable you to get right back onto your plan again. Act out this scenario in your mind. This will enable you to bounce back and get going with minimum bother if in reality the situation arises.

Above all, keep going. You will be successful if you do.

3) Identify obstacles before they occur and put in place strategies to avoid them

Most of us know what our weaknesses are. Many of us find it really hard to overcome them. Part of the solution is recognising your weaknesses. The other part is trying to develop a strategy to overcome this, before you are confronted with the situation.

Your Personal Health Plan gives you instruction as to how to identify your weaknesses or triggers. Think of a strategy which you would use to offset the weakness in each situation and make a note of it next to each. See how when you have your plan on paper how it makes it "real" and therefore easier to implement.

Plan how you will handle each scenario. Take a few minutes in a quiet room with your eyes closed to visualise yourself implementing your strategy and overcoming an obstacle as a result. Feel how good it is to succeed. This will make actually putting your strategy into place much easier when the situation arises.

Food and weight safety net strategies

Can't resist buying sweets, cakes or biscuits when doing your weekly shop?

- Do your shopping straight after a meal so you are not tempted by hunger.
- Plan all your meals for the week before going shopping so that you include plenty of fresh ingredients and so that you know that all of your meals are going to come into your healthy eating plan.
- Write a shopping list based on this and stick to it. This will also save money.

Are you are a snacker or a grazer?

- Do something to take your mind off food: run yourself a bath, go for a brisk walk, phone a friend, engage in a hobby.
- Keep plenty of healthy snacks to hand such as fresh fruit, raw vegetables or a mixture of dried fruit and unsalted nuts. Cereal bars are better than sweets but take care, as many of them are loaded with sugar. Choose the ones that haven't got chocolate or caramel on them. Go for the oaty type, which fill you up for longer. These are good to carry around with you, so you won't be tempted to buy unhealthy nibbles if hunger overtakes you while you are out.
- If you love helping yourself to leftovers, make sure that you put the remainder of the meal straight into the bin so that you are not tempted to graze. If they can be used for the following day's meal, make sure that they are covered and put away so that you cannot see them.

Sugar cravings?

- Always eat 3 meals a day.
- Eat at regular times.
- Include plenty of slow release carbohydrates such as wholemeal bread, pasta, brown rice and potatoes in your meals as they fill you up for longer.

Trouble saying no?

- When you are offered food, practise saying "no thank you" politely but firmly to food that doesn't fit in with your healthy eating plan. You can turn this around to make it more positive by saying "no, but I'd love a glass of water or a cup of tea."

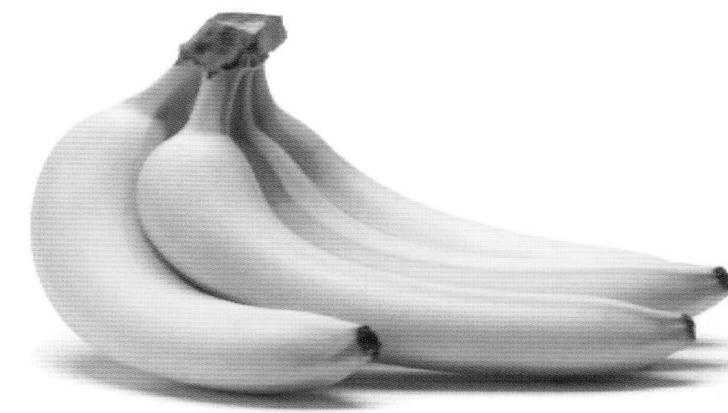

Healthy food beyond your budget?

- Look at the way you shop. Shop, after you have eaten, so you won't be tempted to buy more than you need. Choose store brands as they tend to be cheaper and avoid "buy one get one frees" as they tend to make you buy more than you need. If you write a list before you go and stick to it, this also tends to limit how much you buy.

- Look at the way you eat. Eat a proper breakfast so you are not tempted to buy expensive snacks. Take a packed lunch with you if you go to work, or go out over a meal time. Use tap water, rather than bottled water and if you crave a snack, try a hot drink or brushing your teeth instead. Ready meals tend to be more expensive and are high in fat and sugar anyway so cook all your food from scratch if you can.

- Look at what you eat. The joy of the healthy eating plan is that the mainstay of your diet is made up of slow release carbohydrates like brown bread, pasta and potatoes which are all cheap to buy. Buy your fresh fruit and vegetables when they are in season, they tend to be cheaper. Frozen fruit and vegetables can have just as many vitamins as fresh ones and tend to be cheaper and don't go off, avoiding wastage. Meat and fish can be expensive, and it's not necessary to have this every day. Cook more vegetarian meals.

Large appetite?

- Eat slowly, chewing each mouthful well before swallowing. Aim to be the last one to finish your meal. This works on the principle that when food gets to your small intestine, a hormone is released which tells your appetite centre that you are full. If you rush your food, the body doesn't have time to release the hormone before you have eaten too much.

- Always eat sitting down.

- Drink plenty of water during the meal. It fills you up and also keeps your kidneys healthy. Take care with this one in the evenings if you have an over-active bladder.

- Wait for 5 minutes after finishing your meal before going for a second helping.

- Ask yourself before you take a second helping whether or not you are really still hungry. You will find as you eat less that after a while your stomach will accommodate and a smaller meal will fill you up.

Dr Christian Barnard, the late South African Cardiac surgeon who performed the world's first heart transplant, when asked how he kept himself so trim, replied that his mother taught him as a child to stop eating at a point in the meal before he felt completely full.

"Pain (any pain-emotional or physical) has a message. The information it has about our life can be remarkably specific, but it usually falls into one of two categories: "we would be more alive if we did more of this" and "life would be lovely if we did less of that." Once we get the pain's message and follow its advice, the pain goes away"

Peter McWilliams

A word on comfort eating

If you bottle up your emotions you are not allowing your body to deal with a situation and move on. Many people who try to hide their emotions by pushing them down, in turn use food to push down their emotions. This is comfort eating. The act of comfort eating rarely makes us feel better, because even if the original emotion has been quashed it is often replaced with guilt. Moreover, more often than not, we still have the cause of the original emotion left to deal with.

The healthiest way to deal with emotion is to allow yourself to feel and express it in a controlled fashion. You may want to do this by talking. Sharing a problem with someone else often allows you to see the problem more clearly and even if you don't come up with answers, just "getting it off your chest" can be incredibly therapeutic.

Writing can help; keeping a diary or writing a letter can be a really good way of clarifying your thoughts. If you are really angry, write a letter to the person or organisation that has caused your stress and then burn it. This can be quite cathartic and helps to dissolve your distress. If you decide to send the letter, wait a week before doing so as you may feel differently when you have calmed down.

Exercise can be a really good way of getting rid of stress or anger and also has the benefit of helping your health plan.

It is appropriate if something bad or distressing happens to you that you should be allowed to grieve.

If you are a comfort eater, try and recognise what emotions or situations trigger your eating. Keep a Diet Diary for a week, (see page 133 in your Personal Health Plan) and use this to identify your triggers. Stress and boredom are common causes for comfort eating.

Once you have identified your triggers, put in place a strategy that you can use the next time that situation arises. For instance, if you feel the need to eat a bar of chocolate after every time you speak to a relative who winds you up on the phone, replace this with going to run a long relaxing bath, going for a brisk walk or talking to someone who you feel close to.

Use positive language to dispel any negative feelings. Utilise your visualisation techniques to visualise the positive outcome of your next stressful situation. Remind yourself how well you are doing with something that is going right for you. You may find the relaxation exercise described on page 90 helps to calm you.

If you get stressed about specific things, identify what those stresses are. Write them down and try and work out a strategy for each one. If you feel the need to turn to food when stressed, increase time in your day for yourself to do "you-focused" things (see "Time Management", page 121).

If you are bored, write down why you think you are, and make a positive decision to change something in your life to make it better.

Safety net strategies to increase your exercise level

Trouble getting motivated?

- Extend your Comfort Zone slowly by starting gently. Build your exercise into your normal working routine: take the stairs instead of the lift, walk to work or get off the bus one or two stops early and walk the remainder, walk to the shop to post a letter or buy a paper, rather than drive.

- Practise picturing yourself finishing an exercise session, imagining how good you will feel having done it.

- Alternatively you could engage the support of your partner for emotional support and encouragement, to go for it when you really don't feel like it when you're fed up or stressed (it's usually at these times that you need the exercise most and also at these times that if you didn't you might succumb to comfort eating).

- Start a regime with your partner, whole family or a friend. This is a really good way of keeping your enthusiasm going, until your routine becomes a habit and is incorporated into your Comfort Zone. Once your regime is habit, it is much easier to maintain.

- Remember, use lots of positive language and encouragement with yourself.

- Write down your goal for the week and put it up on the fridge or carry it around with you in your diary. Keep looking at it and reminding yourself as to why you are doing it.

Child care?

- Check out the crèche facilities at your local gym. They may require you to be on site however.

- Many swimming pools have a play pen on the pool-side in which you can leave your baby or toddler while you swim if you are lucky enough to have a placid child.

- If finances allow, you could enlist the help of a child minder a couple of times a week to free up some time for yourself. Many parents feel terribly guilty about leaving their child with someone else so that they can do something pleasurable for themselves. This "you" time is as important for your child as it is for you. You will find yourself coming back refreshed and energised and although the time you spend together may be shorter, its quality will be far greater. It's a win-win situation.

- You could get together with a friend or group of friends and take it in turns to look after each others' children while the other goes and exercises.

- You could alternate with your partner. Perhaps one of you goes football training, for example, while the other looks after the children on one or two nights of the week, while on other nights the other person could go to an exercise class, while their partner does the child care.

- When your children are older, instead of sitting at the pool or pitch side while they do their sport, you could take half an hour to go for a walk or run.

"Walking is good for solving problems-it's like the feet are little psychiatrists"

Pepper Giardino

Trouble with transport?

- Walk or cycle to a venue.
- Consider car sharing (if you join a club where there are regular session times you may be able to enlist the help of someone at the club).
- Use a form of exercise that you can do from home, for example walking, running, cycling.

Difficulty with finance?

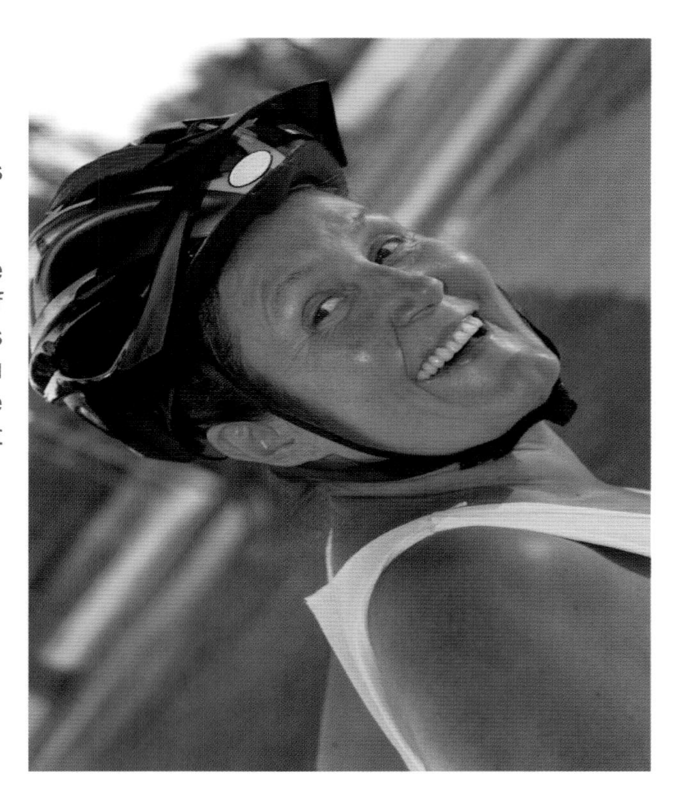

- Consider the more affordable sports such as walking or running.
- Buy a second hand bicycle. The internet has really opened up sale of second hand goods and most sports equipment is available on e-bay. If you don't have a computer, libraries have internet access these days and internet cafés are in most towns.
- Ask your GP about Exercise Referral schemes which at least are cheaper initially.
- Look at council gym membership schemes which are much cheaper than private clubs and gyms.

Poor self confidence?

- Most gyms will put up a list of their quiet times, so that you don't have to attend with the fitness fanatics.
- Check with your local pool when their ladies or men only sessions are.
- Check with your local pool if they offer adult swimming classes.
- Exercise with a friend.
- Exercise at home. There are some really good products on the market for the "home gym". Some are more costly than others. Have you heard of a "Turbo-trainer?" This is a device costing from £50 upwards, that you can clip your bicycle to and can use your cycle indoors or in the garage in a static fashion, in much the same way as an exercise bike. This can keep you fit during the winter, when it is too cold or wet to ride outdoors or if you can't get to the gym.

Smoking Safety net

Challenge frightens you?

- Work out what it is that you're frightened of. Write it down and think of a strategy to get around it. This is all about moving gently out of your Comfort Zone. Often the thought of "the unknown" is far worse than the reality.

- Use positive language to encourage yourself. Practice saying "I am a non smoker" and "no, I don't smoke" politely but firmly.

- Write down 5 good things about being a non smoker and 5 bad things about being a smoker. Pin the list to your fridge.

- Throw away of all your cigarettes and ash trays.

- Get your friends and family on board. Ask your friends who smoke, not to smoke around you. Encourage them to support you.

- Encourage yourself. Congratulate yourself regularly and tell yourself how well you are doing.

- Use all the help that is on offer to you in the form of support clinics, help lines and medication to help with the withdrawal symptoms.

Need to be busy?

- Don't quit on a weekend or while on holiday. Quit at the beginning of a working week, when you will be occupied for much of the time.

- Take up a hobby to occupy your mind and hands.

- Start an exercise regime. This will help keep your weight down and is a great stress buster.

Habit cigarette hard to kick?

- Change your routine. If it's a cigarette in the car, walk to work if it's possible, or share a lift to work with someone who doesn't smoke. Alternatively you could try chewing sugar-free gum in the car.

- If it's a cigarette after an alcoholic drink, avoid the pub for a bit.

- If it's a cigarette with a cup of coffee, try orange juice for a while.

Need to have something in your hand all the time?

- Replace your cigarette with a carrot or celery stick. Cinnamon sticks are really good because you can chew on them and you can also inhale through them.

- Some people find a form of nicotine replacement therapy called an inhalator helpful. It is shaped like a cigarette and you can inhale through it and get a dose of nicotine as you do so. These are available to buy over the counter and on prescription from your GP.

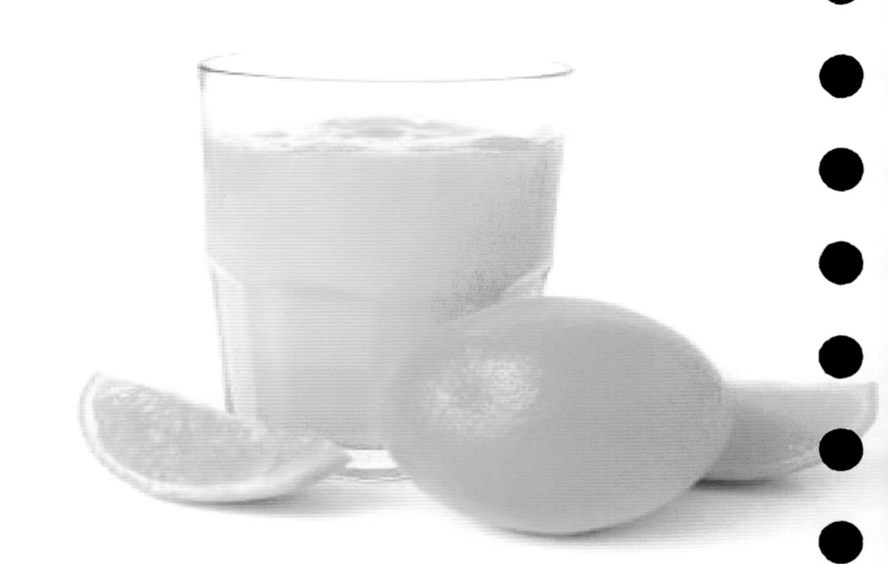

Cravings?

- Use one of the medicines available to help reduce cravings, such as Nicotine Replacement products, Buproprion Hydrochloride or Varenicline. Don't wait until you have cravings. Make sure that you have your choice of product ready before you get to your stop smoking deadline. Some of the products require you to have started them a week or so before hand.

- Remember the huge craving will only last for a few minutes and then will die down. Hang on for those few minutes.

- Distract yourself during this time with a task, a walk, brushing your teeth or healthy snack. Sugar free gum can be helpful.

- Deep relaxation techniques (see page 90) can be really good to carry you over these urges and get easier to do the more you practice them. You can use them at other stressful times.

- Some find relief from cravings using acupuncture or hypnosis. If you consider using one of these techniques, make sure you choose a practitioner who is registered with a professional body. Turn to page 79 for the contact details of The British Complementary Medicine Association and The Institute of Complementary Medicine.

- Remember, the cravings will only last for a few weeks and will become more spaced out. Try not to be taken by surprise by them when they occur out of the blue as they probably will. Have a plan in your mind before this happens as to what you will do when it comes.

Ring:

NHS Smoking Helpline: telephone 0800 169 0 169

Quitline: 0800 00 22 00

"Change your thoughts and you change your world"

Norman Vincent Peale

Alcohol safety net

Hard to say no?

- Practice saying “no” firmly but politely.
- Alternate a non alcoholic or low alcohol drink with an alcoholic one.
- Order drinks with a lower percentage alcohol.
- Drink small measures.

Drink too much?

- Pace yourself. You don’t have to keep up with those around you. If you are with a group buying rounds, skip a round or two. You could create a delay. Go somewhere for five minutes to slow down the pace or to give yourself space to ask, “do I really want a drink right now?”
- Go later to the pub so that you have less time to drink.
- Stop drinking alcohol on weekdays.
- Stop drinking alcohol during the day at work.
- When you are socialising give yourself a window of time in which you will drink.
- Avoid salty snacks. They make you thirsty and you will want to drink more.
- Decrease the number of social activities you do that include alcohol.
- Offer to drive others to a venue, so that you have an excuse not to drink.

Lose track of how much you drink in an evening?

- Count your drinks.
- Don’t top up your drinks. You won’t be able to keep track of how much you have drunk.

Caught up in the "habit drink"?

- Change your routine. Use a different route home that avoids the pub; spend more time with a different set of people who drink less heavily. Breaking your routine will busy your mind and hands and will divert your attentions away from ingrained habits. Take up a new hobby. What about an exercise class that will have the double bonus of contributing to your health plan? It will only take a couple of weeks before your body re-adjusts to the new regime.

- If you drink regularly at home, stop buying alcohol with your weekly shop to ensure that you only have it in the house on a night when you have made a positive decision that you would like a drink. If your partner drinks, try and get them on board with this too.

- Buy half rather than full bottles of wine. In the UK these tend to be disproportionately over-priced, but there are moves afoot to try and reduce the cost. Watch this space.

- Use a small glass. You may only be drinking one glass of wine, but if it's the size of a bucket you may find yourself slipping over the safe limit.

- Avoid buying boxes of wine, as it's difficult to keep track of how much you drink.

- When you have poured yourself a glass of wine, put the bottle back into the cupboard or fridge, out of temptation's way.

- Use a vacuum sealer to make a bottle last several days.

- Find an alternative soft drink that you really like. Drinks with a bit of "bite" can be a really good alcohol substitute. Chilli can cause your body to produce its own morphine-like substances called "endorphins" which can have a similar effect to that of alcohol. Try "Luscombe's Hot Ginger Beer" or adding Worcester sauce to tomato juice.

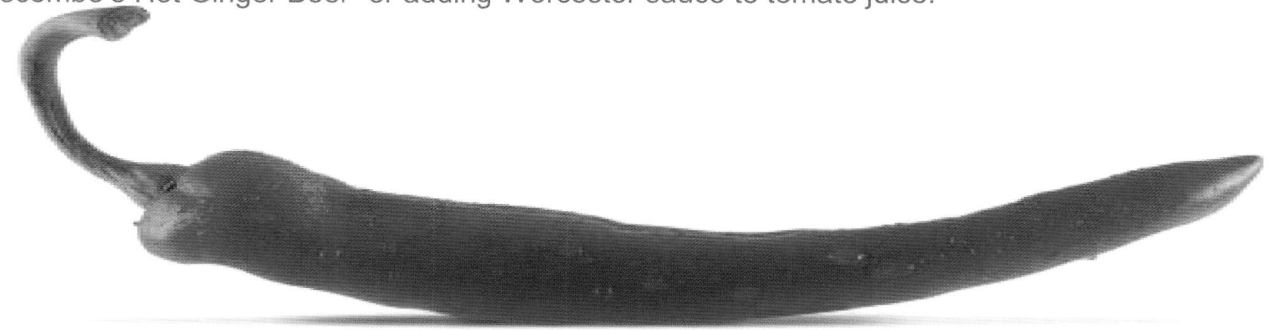

Withdrawal symptoms?

Some of the symptoms experienced could be: severe alcohol cravings, sweating, confusion, agitation, tremor or "shakes."

- Speak to your GP about prescribing something to help.

- Speak to an alcohol counsellor via your GP or using the Alcohol Concern or Alcoholics Anonymous help lines (see page 67 for contact details).

Make a safety net
(Become a black belt in self defence)

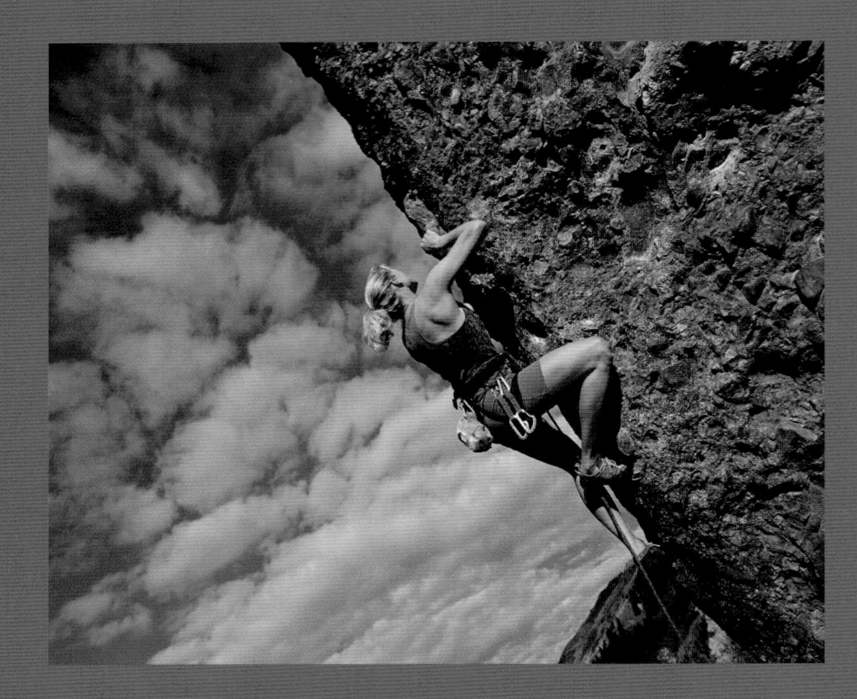

Remember

- Set realistic goals
- Be flexible about set backs; keep going
- Identify obstacles and put in place strategies before you start your programme
- Enlist the support of others

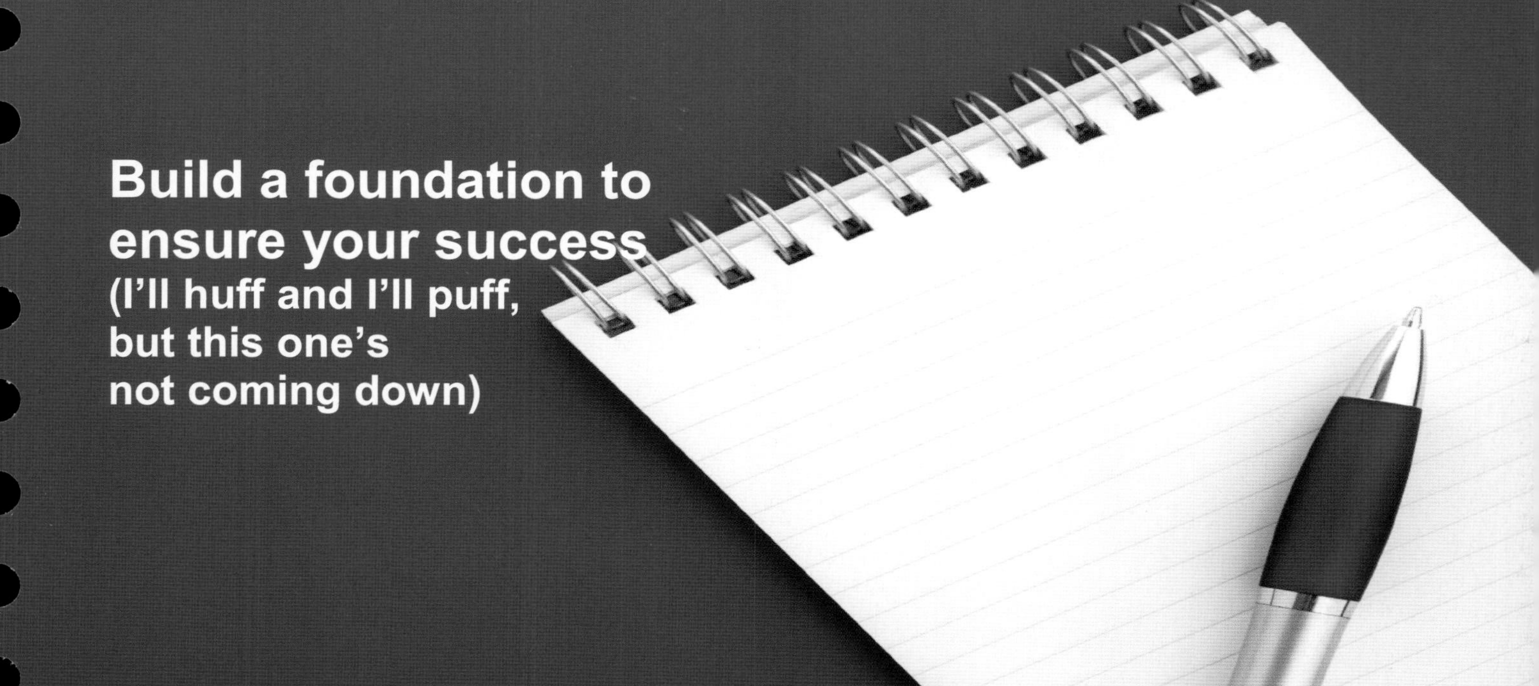

Build a foundation to ensure your success (I'll huff and I'll puff, but this one's not coming down)

In order that you most effectively put your goals into action, you should set up a framework which enables you to carry them out with ease. There are three ways in which you can do this:

- Get active on time management
- Make a team
- Reward yourself

Get active on time management

When I suggest to patients that they incorporate exercise into their routine, the most common reason I hear for not being able to achieve this is time. Many of us lead busy lives, working long hours and juggle family and other commitments alongside this. What we need to do is to somehow make time.

Time management recognises the busy lifestyle and enables you to be able to organise and prioritise to allow you to do all the things that are important and necessary for you to lead a healthy and fulfilled life.

You need to be proactive and to take a step back for a few minutes on a weekly basis, in order to identify what your priorities are. Having taken a few minutes, you will find that a short amount of invested time will open up much more of your week for productive space.

Time management requires you to have the discipline to stick to your priorities, but should also allow you the flexibility to deal with unplanned emergencies. If you can, carry a diary around with you, this will enable you to refer to it easily and amend it if needs be.

You are not required to fill every minute of every day to the exclusion of spending time with your friends and family. In fact what time management does is organises your day in order that you *can* spend time with them, plus doing all the extra things which are important for your health plan. It does however mean that on occasions you will recognise that something is not a priority and you will be able to say "no."

"things that matter most must never be at the mercy of things that matter least"

Goethe

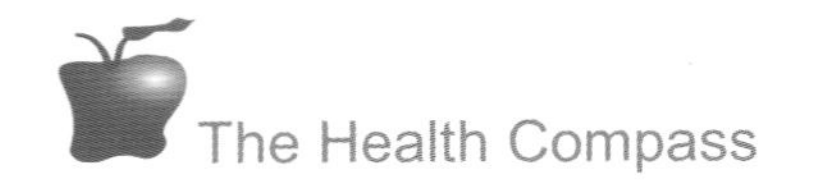

What is the definition of a priority?

A priority is something that should come before all else.

This is a really important concept, as without this, you can't effectively schedule.

A priority is important. However being important doesn't necessarily make something a priority. It is important that I remember to post a package that has to be with a friend in 48 hours, but this is not a priority.

A priority may or not be urgent. When the phone rings, in general it requires my urgent attention but it is only rarely that taking a call on the spot is a priority. If you have had a heart attack however it may be that giving up smoking becomes a matter of both urgency and priority.

A priority is an investment or a building block to your grand plan. An investment is something that will help you achieve your final goals. When planning your week, recognise the difference between important, urgent and priority items. There may of course be some overlap with these things. I find that it's really helpful to have in mind what my current goals are, both long and short term when trying to distinguish between them. I plan around and incorporate both of them, tackling the short term goal with the long term goal as my objective. Your priority items are the ones that definitely need to be slotted in.

It is still important to incorporate your urgent and important items into your weekly schedule. What you will find is if you lay the foundation of a well planned week, you will have the flexibility to deal with important items. You will also have fewer urgent items as you will have dealt with them before they became so.

For instance if I put off renewing the MOT on my car until the day before it expires, it becomes urgent, whereas, if I have the renewal date in my diary at the beginning of the year, with a reminder 2 weeks before the date to organise and book it, it becomes important, but not urgent. If you have lots of urgent items, they take priority in your day and crowd out the opportunity for you to be organising your day in the way that you want. A well planned week should eventually have only a few urgent items. If you do have unplanned emergencies as is inevitable, if you have planned your week sensibly, you will have greater flexibility to deal with them.

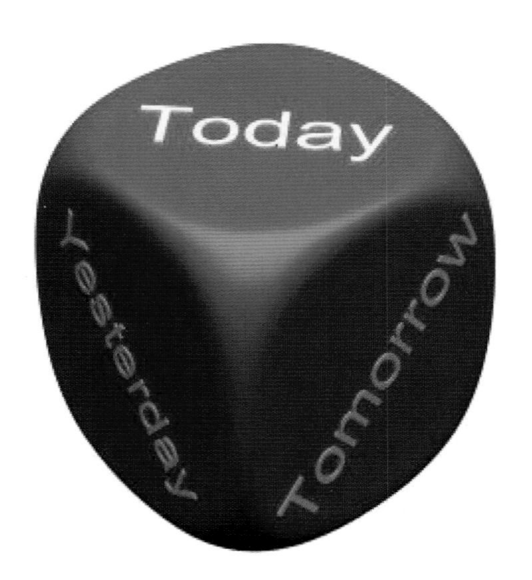

Recognise what isn't a priority. What tasks do you do regularly that you can either say no to or delegate in some way?

Saying "no"

There is nothing wrong with saying "no". Some of us find it really hard to say. This may be because we feel we would cause offence by refusing, or because we feel the need to please other people all of the time. The problem is that saying yes can often be at your own expense of time or energy, you don't have. If you are someone who people always ask to do things because you never refuse, saying no, to start off with will be hard to do, but it does get easier as you do it more.

Make sure that when people make a request of you, don't say yes before you have understood exactly what the request is going to mean for you, in both time and energy. Make sure that you are able to fit the task into your plan. Remember, first things first. Your plan is your investment for you and your family's future. Stick to your plan. If you can, say yes, but if you can't, you have the right to say no.

When saying no, you should be firm but polite. Let the situation decide on your response. You don't have to give a lengthy excuse. You can just say no. Don't make up excuses, because the person will usually know that you are being creative with the truth.

Here are a few ideas of things that you can say to make your response seem more positive:

No, I'd love to help but:

- I've got far too much on at the moment
- I am not taking on any new responsibilities
- I'm not comfortable with that
- I have another commitment
- I have no experience with that
- I need to focus on my career
- I need to focus more on my personal life
- I need to leave some time free for myself
- Sorry I can't help, but I can find you someone who can

Or if you can't avoid saying yes, then make sure you set some boundaries. Here are some ideas:

Agree, but put a proviso on it, for example:

- I'd love to do it, but I can only fit it in next week
- I'd love to help, but I can only spare a couple of hours
- I can help you with this, if you could give me a hand with something else
- I'll help you out on this occasion, but we're going to have to work out a plan so this situation doesn't arise another time

Make a plan

I find the easiest way to plan is to think in weekly chunks. Having a largish diary which shows a week at a time is really useful for this. Taking life a day at a time doesn't give you flexibility and 2 week chunks mean that you have to think too far ahead and end up making loads of changes. Take a few minutes out, on a Sunday, before the start of the next working week, so that you can schedule in all the fixed appointments of the week and from there work around them. I do this in conjunction with my husband, so that I can allow for his work, health and leisure commitments when I am planning my week.

In order to plan your week effectively, break the process down:

1) Identify your roles

Think for a few moments. Try to visualise what your roles are; you will have several. For instance: individual (this would be the place in which you would think of your health goals), husband/wife/partner, son/daughter, mother/father, neighbour, work colleague, committee member or parishioner, for example. Think about what you need to do to fulfil each of these roles over the next week.

2) Set your goals

When you have thought about how you would like to spend your next week in each of your roles, make a list of two or three things for each of those roles that you would like to or need to achieve. You don't have to think long term, although having your long term goal in mind is helpful.

3) Plan your week

If you live on your own, this is a bit simpler. If you have family, you will need to incorporate their schedule into yours. If you take a step back from the bustle of life as it happens, you can see openings and cracks in time which are easy to use, which you perhaps would not have identified otherwise.

Start with putting in all your fixed appointments and commitments, such as work, meetings, and your children's or partner's clubs and activities.

Now look at your goals for the week and schedule them in around your fixed appointments. You may find that you want to list your health/exercise sessions as fixed appointments, so that they never get missed. If you need flexibility in your plan and have the time and capacity to juggle things around, then you can work your health/exercise plan in around your fixed schedule. Once you have completed your plan, you can transfer it into your weekly diary.

Be prepared to adapt your diary on a daily basis.

Check your diary at the beginning of each day. It is inevitable that unplanned and important things will arise. If you have your diary to hand, you can reschedule effectively.

How to fill in your weekly plan

After trying lots of different ways of keeping track of day to day family life, I have found a weekly plan (adapted from Stephen R. Covey, the 7 Habits of Highly Effective People) to be the most effective. You can use this on its own or as the basis for filling in your weekly diary.

On the following page I have taken a week out of the life of Hannah, a working mum, to show you how you might fill it in.

Notice how Hannah has colour coded each of her roles and goals to make it easier to follow her plan. She starts by putting her and her family's fixed commitments on the plan in black and then adds her flexible commitments in colour afterwards.

This is an example of one week, but of course it varies, depending on her flexible commitments. For example, on weeks where Hannah does not have a lunchtime meeting on a Monday, she goes for a swim which frees her up time to spend with her children in the evening.

When her children Jack and Chloe are at dancing lessons on a Friday, Hannah walks the dog, to create time during the day for her to have a drink with a friend or to get some of her household tasks done. She also walks the children home from school with the dog on occasions, for the same reason, and this also gives the children a bit of exercise.

When Hannah's children are at Running Club on Saturday morning she either joins in with them or goes for a run or cycle on her own. This gives her husband, Sam a bit of peace and quiet at home, or time to go back into work to finish off any loose ends.

One of the strengths in Hannah's exercise regime is that she enjoys several different forms of exercise, which makes her much more flexible in what she can achieve. For instance, on a rainy day or in the winter she might choose to swim instead of cycle. On a day when she has to work an extra session, instead of a lunchtime swim, she might do an evening Pilates session instead.

Hannah works a 22 hour week and manages to get in 5 or 6 exercise sessions a week, plus walking the dog 6 days a week. Her husband works a sixty hour week and still manages to get in 4 or 5 exercise sessions a week. They can only do this by thinking ahead and careful planning.

A friend looked at Hannah's weekly plan and commented on how "frenzied" it looked. Hannah obviously thrives on filling every moment. Your plan needs to suit your needs and personality. Everyone is different. You may decide to fill a space with space. That's great. The only thing that is important is that when you have time, you are doing what *you* want with it.

Weekly planner		Weekly Activity Planner Appointments and Commitments						
Roles	**Goals**	**Monday**	**Tuesday**	**Wednesday**	**Thursday**	**Friday**	**Saturday**	**Sunday**
Wife/mother/ dog walker	1) Lucy/Dan for tea 2) Sort out holiday 3) Get Jack's guitar book 4) Book car MOT 5) Walk dog	8am	8am	8am	8am	8am	8am	8am
		9 5) Walk dog	9 Hannah to work all day	9 4) Book car MOT	9) Hannah to work all day	9 7) Health project	9 11) Running club	9
		10 2) Sort out holiday	10	10 10) Cycle with Lara	10	10 7) Health project	10	10
Work	6) Lunch meeting 7) Health project	11 7) Health project	11	11 "	11	11 7) Health project	11	11 5) dog walk with family
		12 7) Health project	12	12	12	12 7) Health project	12	12
		1pm 6) Lunch meeting	1pm	1pm 5) Walk dog with Sam	1pm	1pm 9) Swim	1pm	1pm
		2 3)Get Jack's guitar book	2	2 13) Take JB thanks	2	2 12) See Clare	2	2
Health	8) Pilates 9) Swim 10) Cycle 11) Run	3	3	3	3	3	3 5) Dog walk with family	3
		4 Jack football	4 Chloe netball	4 1)Lucy/Dan for tea	4	4 Kids Dance lessons	4	4 8) Family Tae Kwon-do
		5	5 Jack swimming	5	5	5 5) Dog walk	5	5
		6	6	6	6	6	6	6
Individual development	12) See Clare 13) Take JB thanks 14) Call Jo 15) Call Steve 16) Supper Jo and Tracey	7 Sam football	7	7 Chloe Swim Club	7 8) Hannah Pilates	7	7	7
		8pm 8) Hannah Pilates	8pm 14)Call Jo 15) Call Steve	8pm Sam football	8pm	8pm	8pm 16)supper Jo and Tracey	8pm
		9	9	9	9	9	9	9

Make a team

This is really important. It is very difficult to be consistent or to maintain motivation if your partner, family or friends are not on board.

If you want to improve your diet, it's far easier if you do this as a family. Alternatively if you live alone, start a healthy eating group at work or join a healthy lifestyle group.

If you want to stop smoking or cut down on your alcohol consumption and yet you have a partner who smokes or drinks heavily, or are part of a social group in which smoking and drinking heavily are important, it is much harder to do. You may find that initially, when you are starting to make healthy changes that altering your routine to spend time away from temptation is helpful. Alternatively you could encourage someone close to you to make changes with you. You don't have to exclude yourself from a group, but having someone who is supporting you from within can be really helpful. Even if you can't get them to make the same changes as you, they can encourage you. Having seen you succeeding, they may well be tempted to follow.

If you want to introduce exercise into your life, even if it's simply to encourage you to get out of the door to exercise when your motivation is flagging, your team is essential. If you do long days at work, consider exercising during your lunch break or asking your boss if you can be flexible with your working hours and start or finish a little later on some days. You may be able to get a work colleague to cover you for an hour while you go for a run, swim or walk and then do the same for them on a different day.

It has become the trend not to have a lunch hour. Many people eat on the go and don't have a proper break. Not only is this poor for your digestion, but it doesn't give you the time to emotionally recharge. Having had a lunch break, refreshed, you will be far more productive for an afternoon of work.

Some feel that taking a break, when none of their colleagues do, would breed resentment. Keep in mind your priority that your health is paramount. Consider getting a group of colleagues together to form a lunch time exercise group. Not only will you be more productive as a group, but such arrangements can be great for team building.

My team is my family; my husband who looks after our children for me on the nights that I do Tae Kwondo on my own, and my children who come to Tae Kwondo with me. I, in turn, am an essential part of their team, looking after the children on my husband's squash nights and taking the children to their football, swimming and dancing lessons. Occasionally I enlist the help of a neighbour to sit with the children for half an hour if I need to go out to an evening session and my husband isn't back from work yet.

My husband, my 11 year old daughter and myself all cook. Cooking with your children is a great way of introducing an essential life skill, is fun, bonding and can give them healthy ideas about food. On a day when I am pushed, my daughter will sometimes help me out with the cooking.

We all need each other. Not only is that helpful in practical terms but gives all of us a feeling of great self worth.

"No one can whistle a symphony. It takes a whole orchestra to play it"
H.E. Luccock

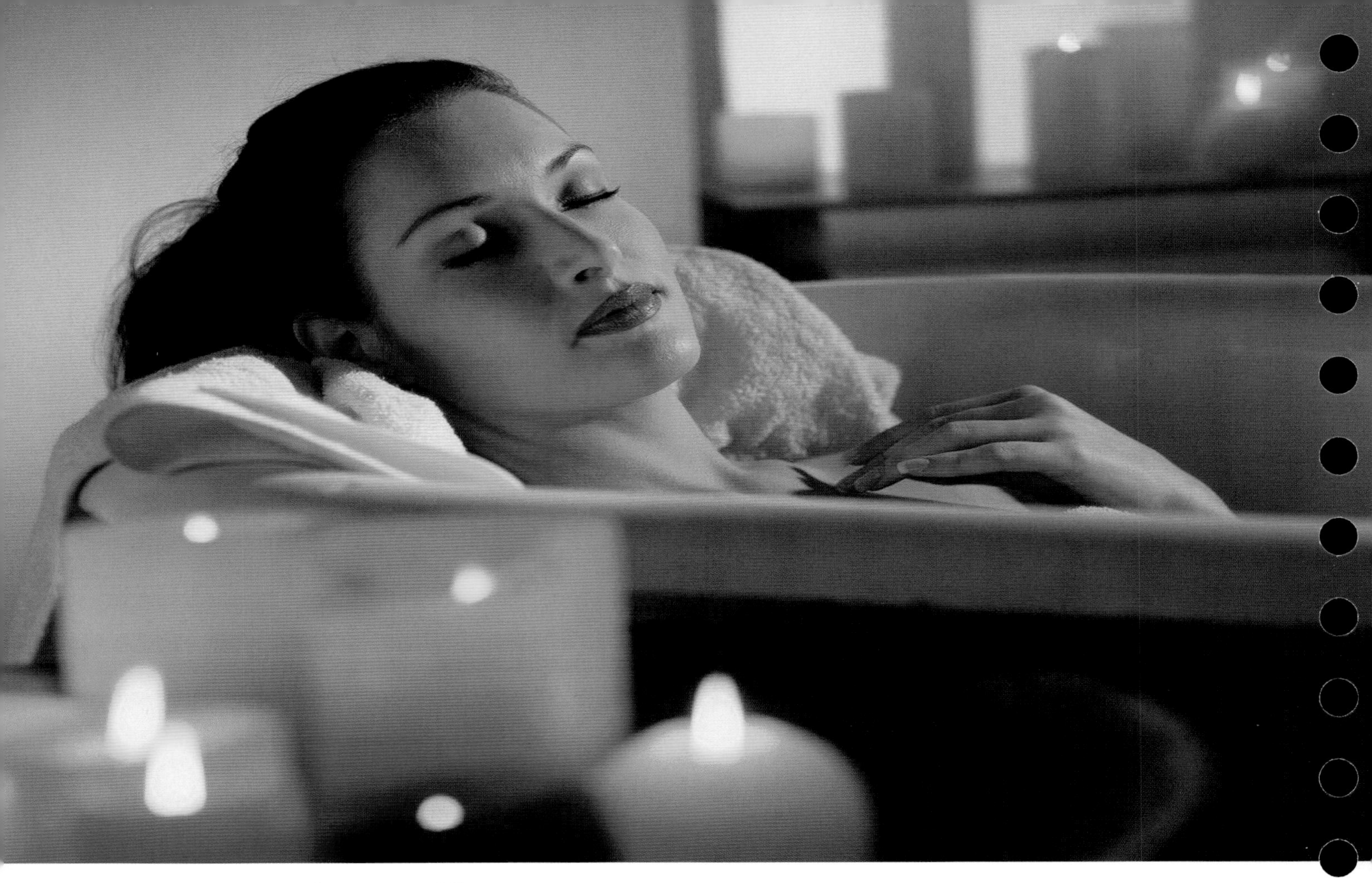

Reward yourself

This is the good one. This is all about recognising your success and congratulating yourself. Make sure when you set your goal that you know what your reward is going to be, as this will give you something to aim for. This is another good reason for setting lots of small goals, rather than one big one. You get to have far more treats!

Preferably, your reward should be something that doesn't work against your lifestyle plan. What do I mean by this? Well, it's ok to do something entirely different from your plan, for example, have a cup of coffee with a friend, have a night out with the boys (staying within your safe alcohol limits of course!), have a long hot bath, go and get your hair done, or go on a shopping trip, as although these things are not part of a healthy living plan, they are not bad for you.

What you need to avoid is congratulating yourself on losing a stone by buying a large cream cake, or allowing yourself a cigarette, to say well done for not having smoked for the last month!

Get a jar and keep the money you have saved when giving up smoking or cutting down on your alcoholic drinks. You can spend it on something you really want. If you smoke 20 a day, £2000, saved over a year, could buy you a holiday or you could get something done on your house. If you are on a low budget it could buy you sports equipment or help fund your healthy eating plan.

If your partner or family have helped in your achievements, remember to reward them too. They are your team. You need to keep it strong.

Remember if you are rewarding someone else, to bear in mind what they would enjoy, not what *you* think they should. A friend of mine, described trying to reward her daughter with a day out walking, because that was what she enjoyed, when all her daughter wanted was to have her hair highlighted.

Build a foundation to ensure your success
(I'll huff and I'll puff, but this one's not coming down)

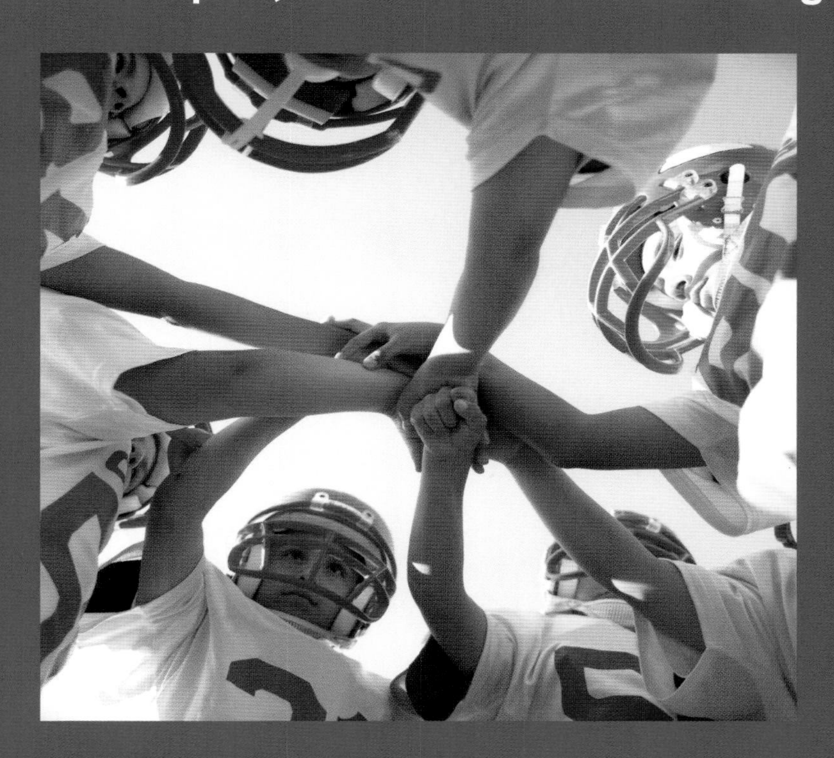

Remember

- Work on your time management
- Sort out your priorities
- Delegate or say no to things that you can
- Use a weekly planner
- Make a team
- Reward your successes; you deserve it

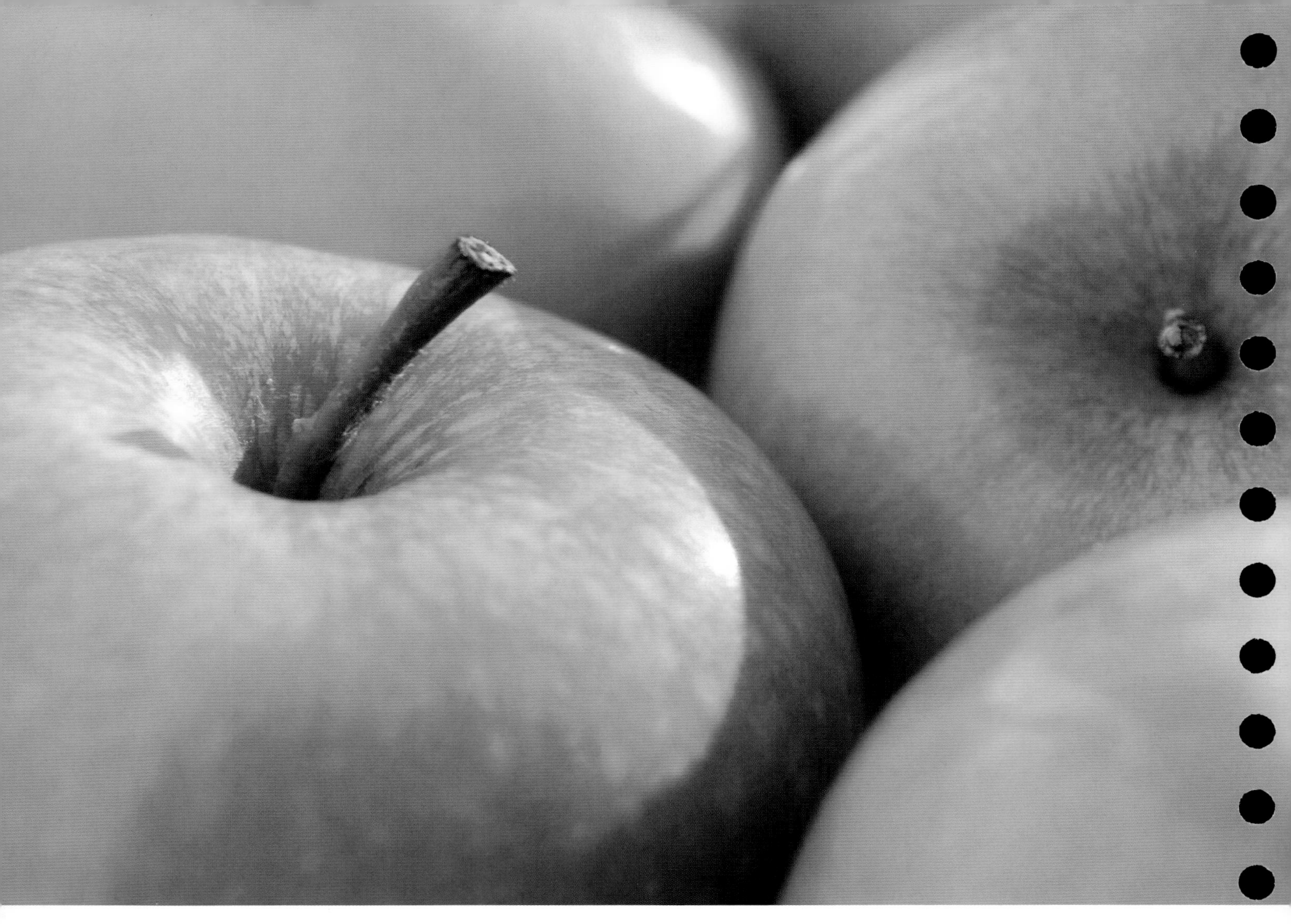

Congratulations

You should now be ready to put into practice what you have learned.

In Parts One and Two, I have shown you the basics of what you need to lead a healthy life. I have given you the tools that you need to put that into practice. All that remains is for you to get started.

Remember, it is much better to start small and keep this going for good, than to go for bust in a way that you are unable to maintain.

Pace yourself. Small steps lead to great things. Remember, this is about a lifetime of change. It maybe that the time is not right for you to be able to do everything you ideally would like at this stage. What is important is that you lay the foundations for when you are able to make bigger changes. Having a few basics in place will make it much easier to achieve better things at a later date.

Focus on your own goals. Don't be distracted by anyone else's. By all means plan and work with someone else. In fact most people find it more supportive and fun to do this. It is by far the best way forward. However, realise that whoever you are working with will almost definitely work at a different pace to you, whether it be faster or slower. Keep pace with yourself and not them.

Encourage yourself and others and celebrate both your and their success

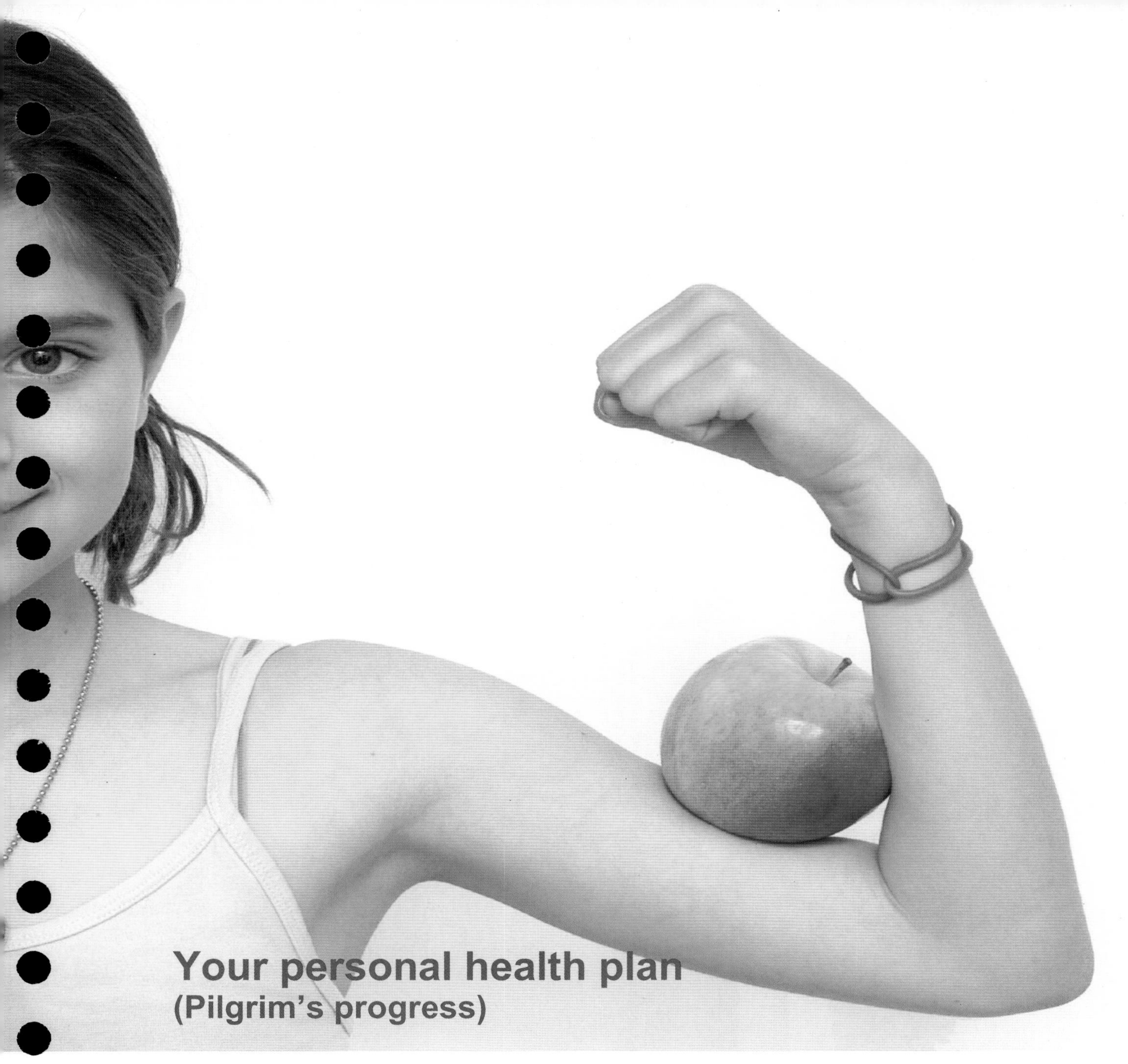

Your personal health plan
(Pilgrim's progress)

Let me introduce you to your Personal Health Plan. You are about to launch on a lifetime of great changes. You will see, that with the knowledge that you have accumulated about what constitutes a healthy lifestyle and how to include these changes in your life, that it really is easy to do, once you have the right framework to build on.

Your Personal Health Plan is the starting point. It marks where you are now and gives you a base from which to spring. Take the area which interests you most and use all the tools you have learned: visualisation, positive language, deep relaxation, goal setting, safety netting, time management, team building and reward. These techniques will allow you to cement your changes firmly into your life.

As you are successful in one area, you will feel your confidence grow and you can tackle another. Making a record in your Personal Health Plan will make it easier to reach your goals and will allow you to return to your starting point, to see just how much you have achieved.

Welcome to the start of your new healthy life

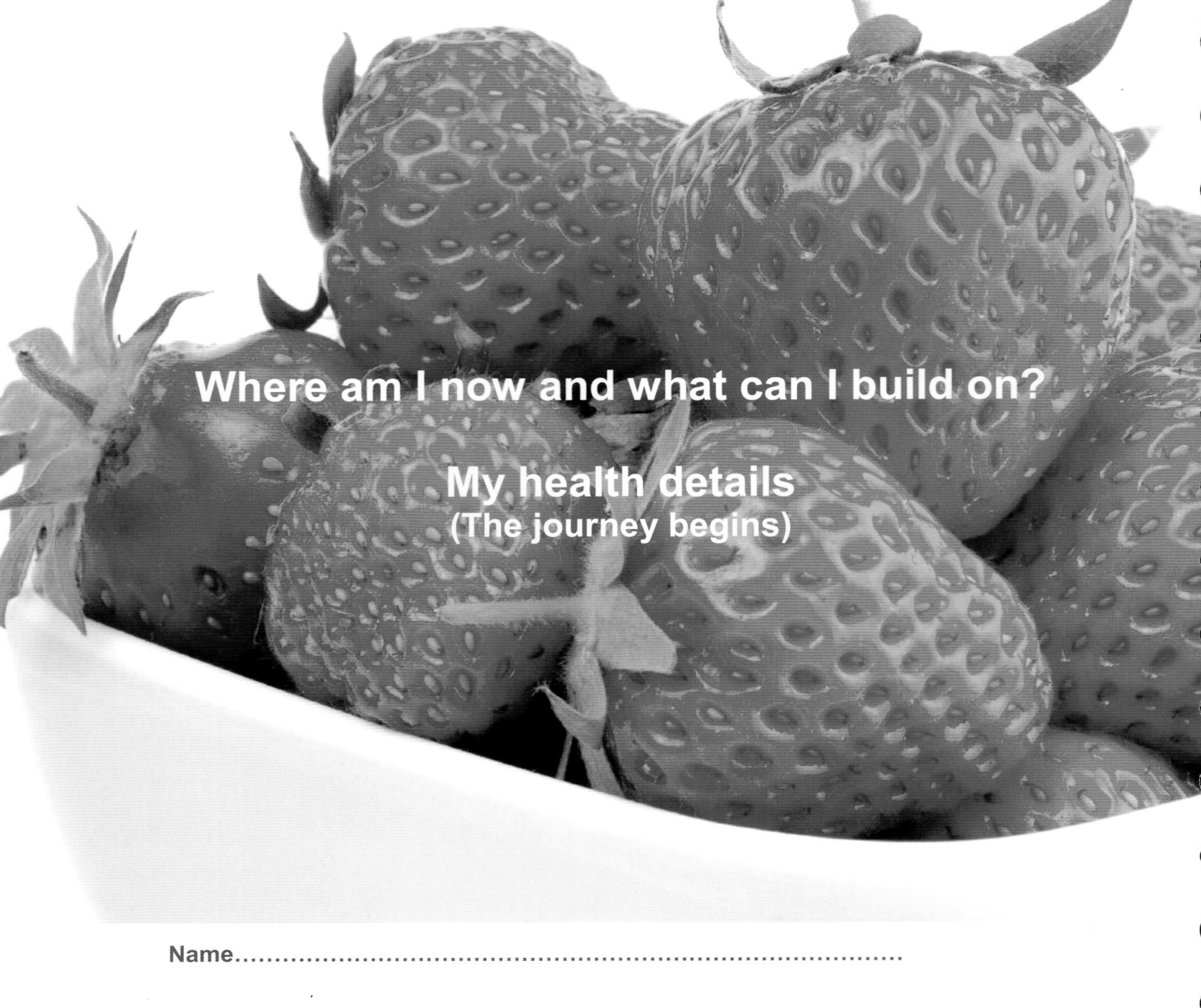

Where am I now and what can I build on?

My health details
(The journey begins)

Name...

Weight..

Height..

BMI..

Ideal weight...

Blood pressure...

Units of alcohol drunk per week.......................................

Number cigarettes smoked per day....................................

 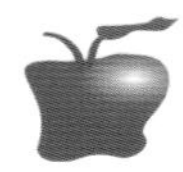

My diet diary
(Strawberry fields forever)

Make a note of everything you eat during the course of a week, writing down the time at which you ate and the circumstances; who you were with and what you were doing. Having done this you will be able to build up a picture of what your triggers are. That is what it is that makes you want to eat. Include snacks and both soft and alcoholic drinks, recording the number of teaspoons of sugar you have in hot drinks.

Monday
Tuesday
Wednesday
Thursday
Friday
Saturday
Sunday

"We are indeed much more than what we eat, but what we eat can nevertheless help us to be much more than what we are"

Adelle Davis

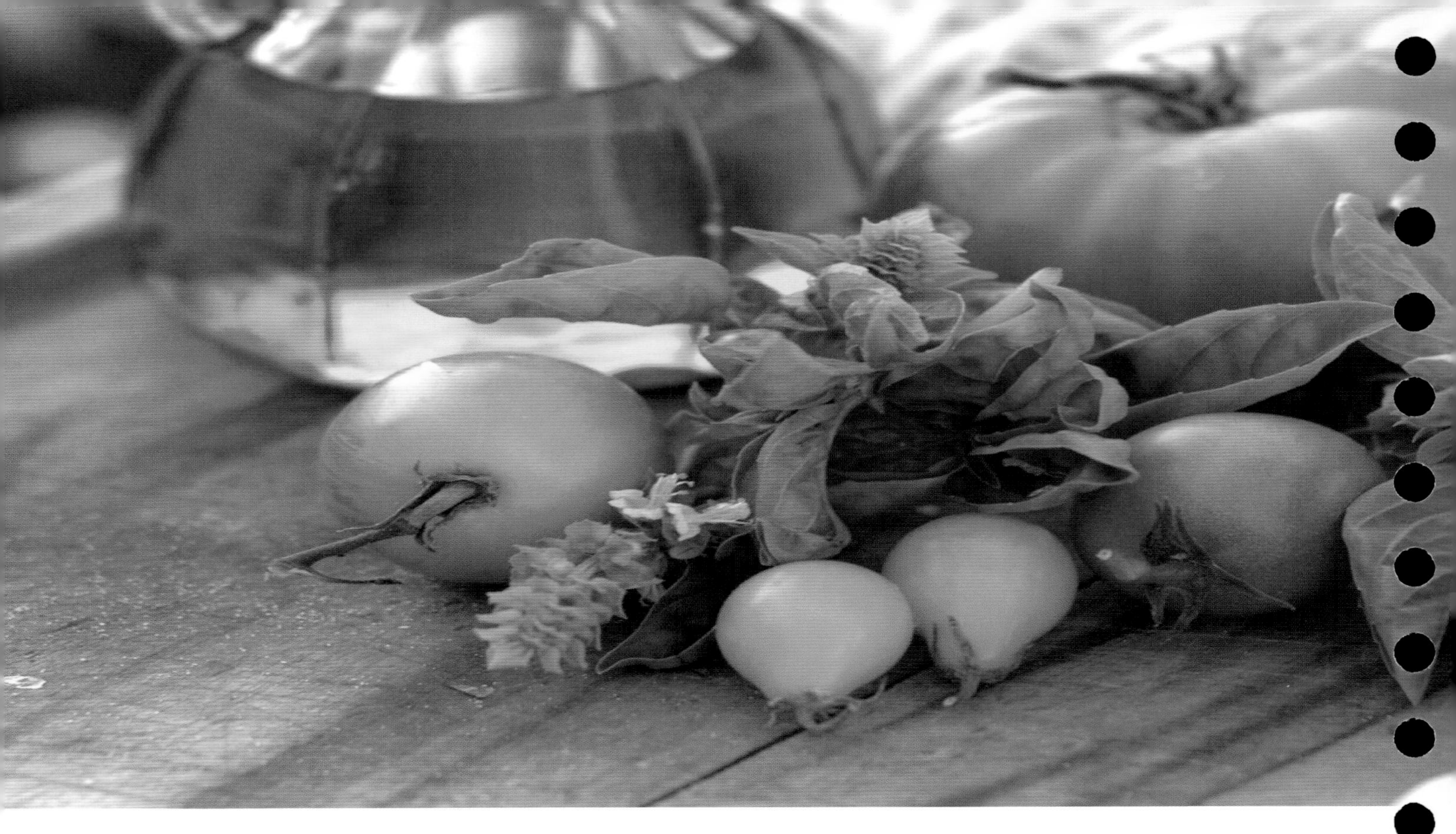

At the end of a week of keeping a Diet Diary, use the check list below to look at how many portions of the different food groups you have used and compare it to the recommended daily allowances. You can use this to plan your healthy eating regime.

Recommended number of portions per week	**Number of portions per week that I have had**
Fruit and vegetables: 35 portions	
Bread, cereals, potatoes, rice and pasta: 49-56 portions	
Milk and dairy (low fat if possible): 14-21 portions	
Meat, fish and eggs: 14-21 portions	
Fatty foods, including crisps and chips: 7-14 portions	
Sugary foods, including sweets, chocolate, biscuits, cakes and sugary or alcoholic drinks:7 portions	

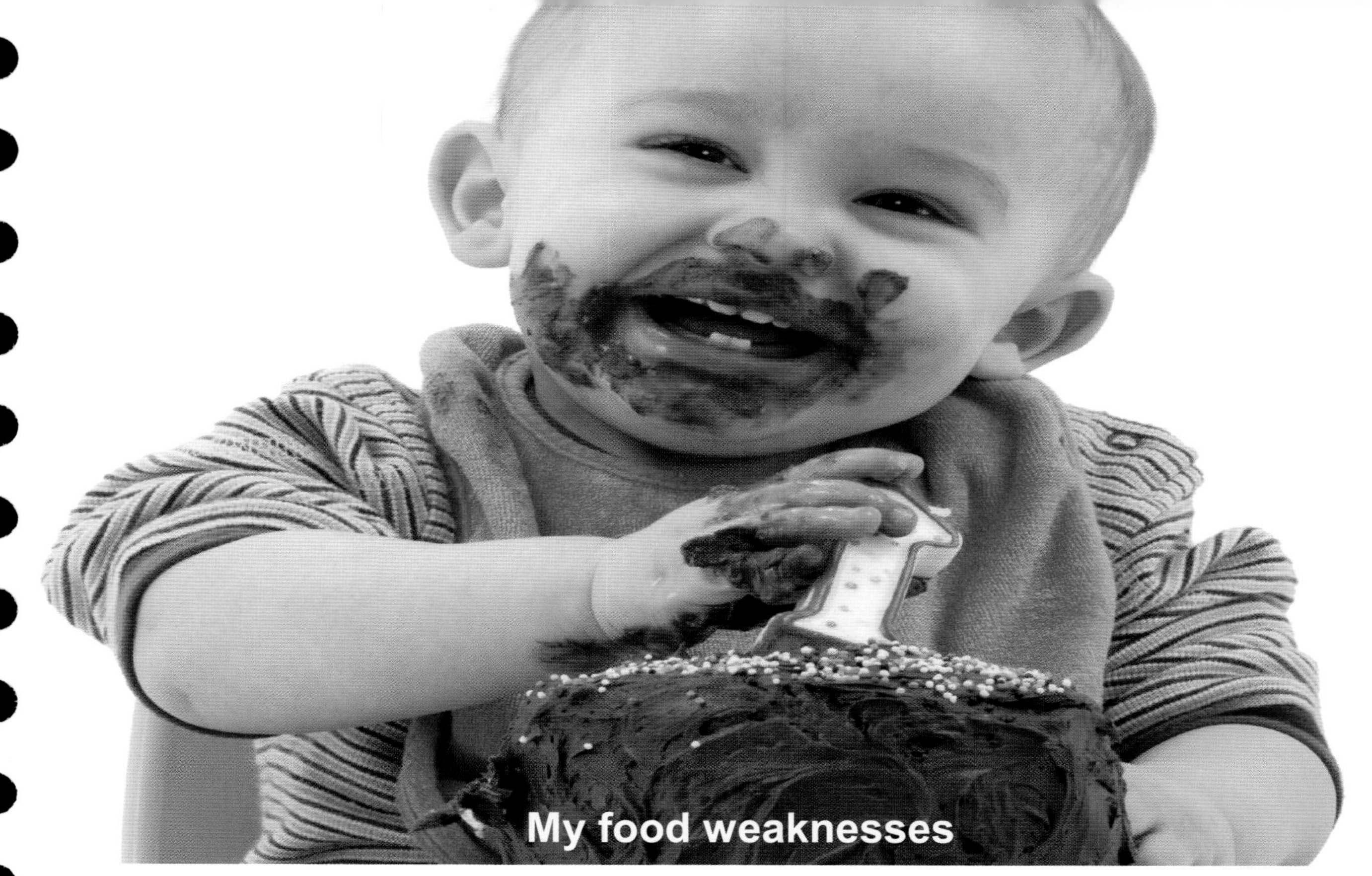

My food weaknesses

Record your weaknesses below (eg grazing, snacking, portion size, skipping meals then bingeing, too many sweet things, fatty foods, fizzy drinks, sugar in tea or coffee, ready made meals or too much salt).

Now you have identified your weaknesses, next to each one on your list, write down a strategy that you can use to tackle it. Use this plan in the next section when you are setting your goals. Keep this log and return to it in three months and repeat it, to see how your regime has improved. Coming back to this can be an ongoing part of your dietary planning.

My food weaknesses	Strategies

My exercise diary
(A little less conversation, a little more action)

The recommended level of exercise is 30 minutes 5 times a week. Are you achieving this regularly? Use the table below to record the exercise you do over the course of a week. Compare that to the recommended level. Remember, some domestic tasks, if done at a vigorous enough level can count.

Day
Monday
Tuesday
Wednesday
Thursday
Friday
Saturday
Sunday

How to create your own exercise plan

Use the information you have gathered to help plan your new exercise regime. You don't have to go for the recommended level straight away. Build things up gradually and get used to one stage at a time. Remember, this is a regime that you will be keeping going for life, so it must be one you can maintain.

Plan and execute your regime, using strategies such as visualisation, positive thinking, goal setting, safety netting, time management, team building and reward.

Remember, reward yourself with things that don't work against your healthy lifestyle plan.

Use the "my goal" page to work out how you will gradually introduce and build on your exercise regime. Then record your progress overleaf.

Include how long you exercised for, what you did in that time and how you felt at the end of it.

It's helpful to come back to this in three months time to see how far you have progressed. I have started off with a 4 week plan. You can keep this going in a separate diary if you want when this has finished.

"My grandmother started walking 5 miles a day when she was 60. She's 93 today and we don't know where the hell she is"

Ellen DeGeneres

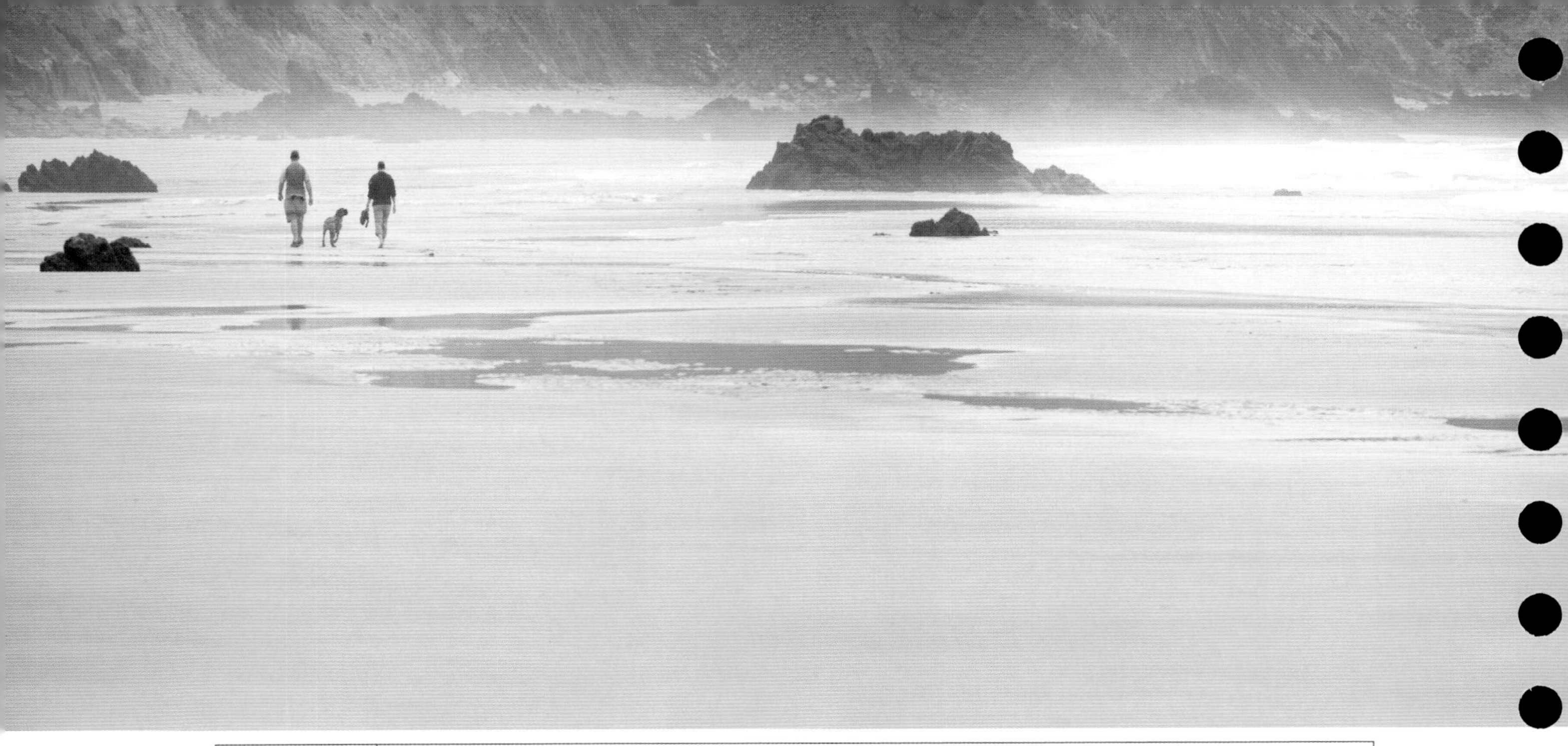

Date	My exercise diary

Date	

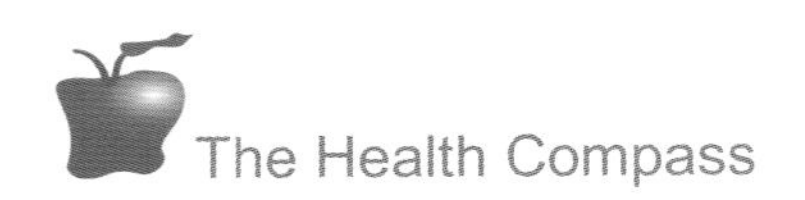

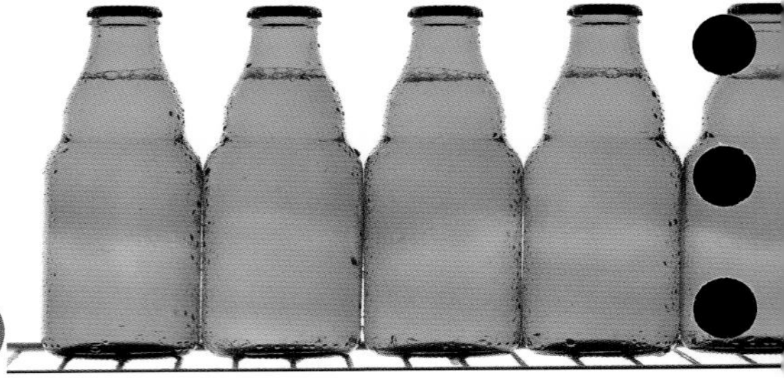

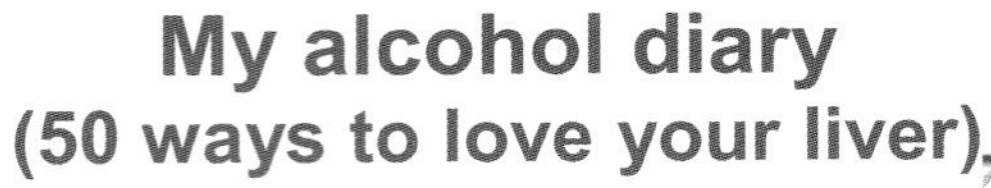

My alcohol diary
(50 ways to love your liver)

Record your alcohol consumption every day for a week. Remember, be honest. Make a note of all alcoholic drinks. Record where you were and who you were with to get some idea of what your triggers are. From here you can work out some strategies to help reduce your consumption.

Day	What	Where/when/who with	Units	Total
Monday				
Tuesday				
Wednesday				
Thursday				
Friday				
Saturday				
Sunday				
		Total units of alcohol for the week		

The recommended safe upper limit of alcohol consumption for adults in the UK is 21 units a week for men and 14 units a week for women

My alcohol triggers

With the information gathered from your alcohol diary, use the space below to make a note of your alcohol triggers. Next to each one write a strategy that you might use to help overcome or avoid that trigger. You can use some of the ideas in the "safety netting" section of Part Two. You can also draw on the other tools in this section such as visualisation, positive thinking and goal setting.

My alcohol triggers	Strategies

Reasons for reducing my alcohol consumption

Below, list your reasons for reducing your alcohol intake. You can pin it up somewhere prominent or carry it around with you to motivate you.

The Fagerström test for nicotine dependence
(No smoke without fire)

This short questionnaire will give you some idea as to how dependent you are on nicotine. This is the questionnaire that stop smoking professionals use to assess what dose of nicotine replacement you need.

Questions	Answers	Points
1) How soon after you wake up do you smoke your first cigarette?	Within 5 minutes	3
	Within 6-30 minutes	2
	Within 31-60 minutes	1
	After 60 minutes	0
2) Do you find it difficult to refrain from smoking in places where it is forbidden for example in church, at the library or cinema?	Yes	1
	No	0
3) Which cigarette would you hate most to give up?	First one in the morning	1
	All others	0
4) How many cigarettes do you smoke?	10 or less	0
	11-20	1
	21-30	2
	31 or more	3
5) Do you smoke more frequently in the first few hours after waking than during the rest of the day?	Yes	1
	No	0
6) Do you smoke when you are so ill that you are in bed most of the day?	Yes	1
	No	0
	Total score	

Low dependency	**1-3**
Moderate dependency	**4-6**
High dependency	**7-10**

My motivation for stopping smoking

Use the space below to write down 5 reasons why smoking is bad for you and another 5 reasons why stopping smoking will be good for you. Use the section on vision (page 144) and goals (page 147) to make a plan of how you will go about stopping. Draw on all resources discussed in Part Two of the book, including visualisation, positive thinking, goal setting, safety netting, team building and reward. Use all help that is available in the form of clinics/quit lines/web sites/medication.

Reasons why smoking is bad for me	Reasons why stopping smoking is good for me

My smoking triggers

Write down your smoking triggers. That is, the things that make you want to light up a cigarette. Take a look at the section on "safety netting" for some ideas on strategies that you might use to help avoid falling into the trigger trap. Make sure you do this exercise before you quit so that you have a good idea of your strategies and have practiced them in your mind. You can use the visualisation/relaxation exercise in Section Two to help.

My smoking triggers	Strategy

Lifestyle toolkit
(Highway to health)

The following section (page 144-156) gives you the framework to put all you have learned from your diet/exercise/alcohol and smoking diaries into practice. Have fun.

My vision

Remember

Always keep your ideas and vision positive. Try and use images and thoughts that will help with your health plan. Imagine how you will feel when you achieve your dream. Use the deep relaxation exercise to help reinforce your vision. If you find yourself slipping into negative thinking, you have the power to block those thoughts and convert them into positive ones.

Use this space to record your vision.

"You see things and you say "Why?" but I dream of things that never were and say "Why not?"

George Bernard Shaw

Page for positive thoughts

Things to include

Write down five positive things about yourself. Using your vision as an aid, write down some positive things that might help you achieve your vision. Avoid using the word "try" and replace it with "will"

For example: I will give up smoking
I am strong
I have the power to change my life

"Reflecting on how we think is one of the most powerful ways we can take more control over our lives"

Paul McGee

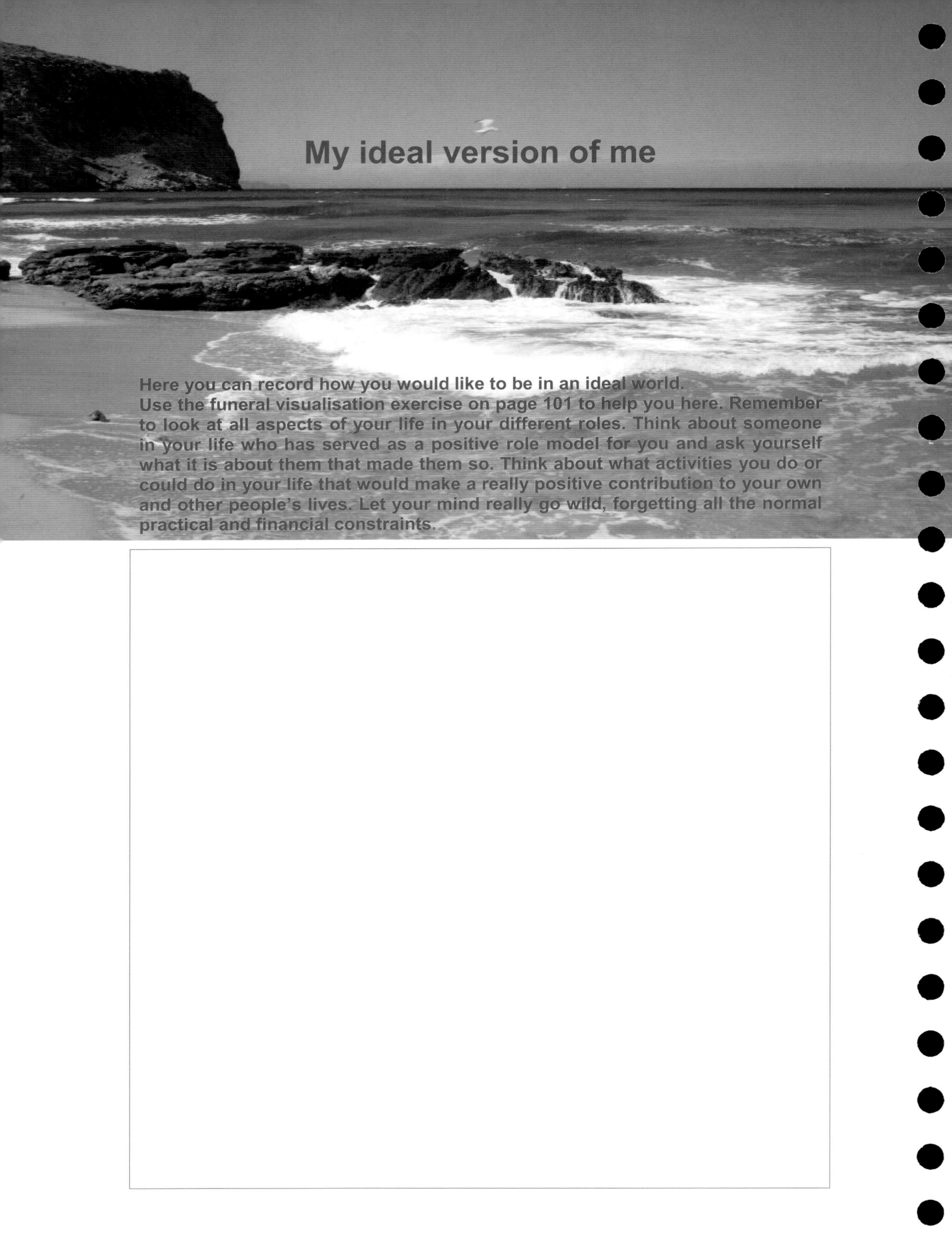

My ideal version of me

Here you can record how you would like to be in an ideal world.
Use the funeral visualisation exercise on page 101 to help you here. Remember to look at all aspects of your life in your different roles. Think about someone in your life who has served as a positive role model for you and ask yourself what it is about them that made them so. Think about what activities you do or could do in your life that would make a really positive contribution to your own and other people's lives. Let your mind really go wild, forgetting all the normal practical and financial constraints.

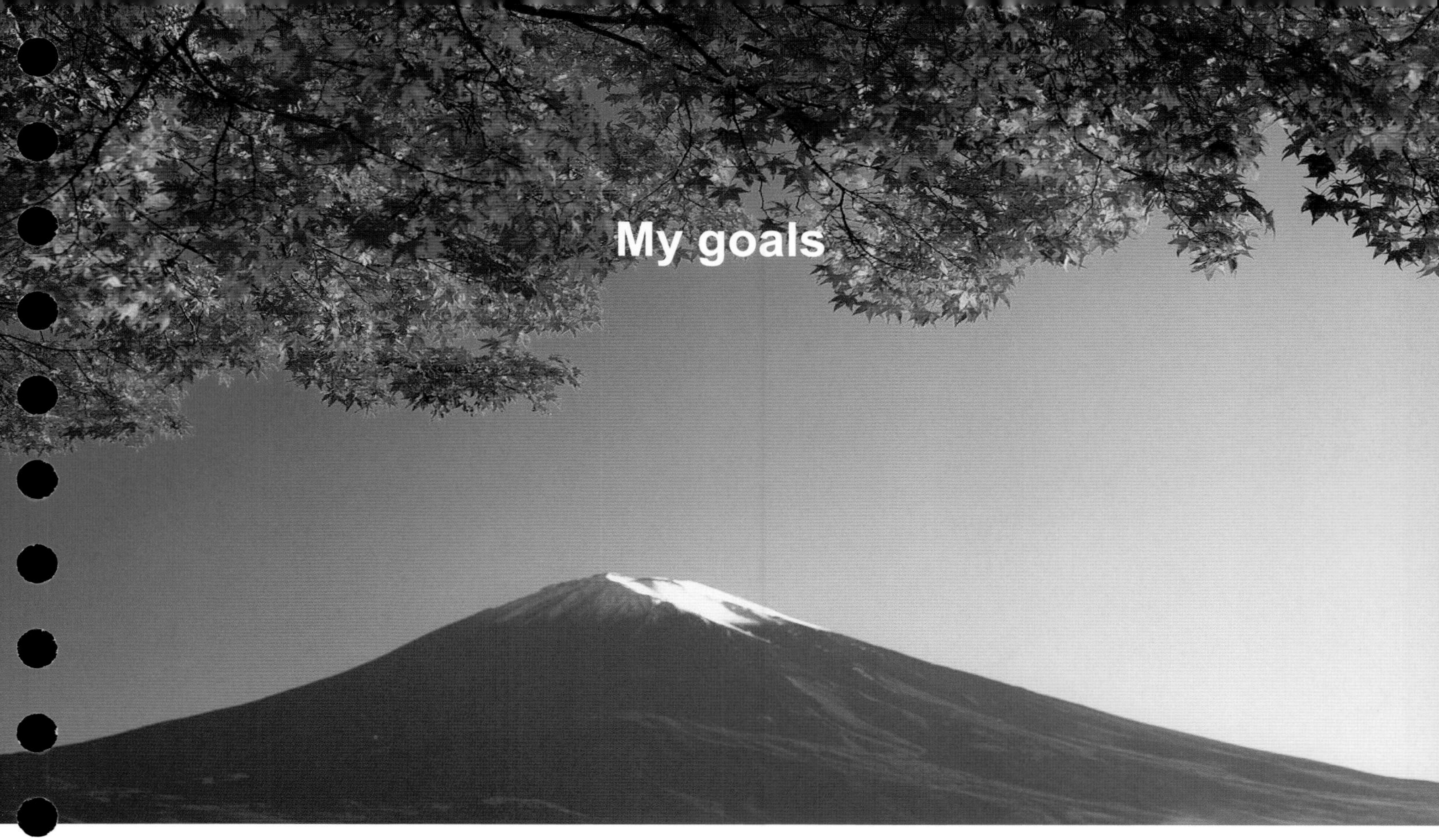

My goals

This section is for your goals. Remember to look ahead to the next 5 years or beyond for your long term goals. This is the direction that you will use your medium and short term goals to take you in. For the purposes of this book you should try and make the focus of your goal a health related one, however, you can use this for all aspects of your life. Notice how much more space I have left you to record your short term goals. That is because I want you to break down each of your goals into bite sized pieces. You should have many small goals. This will make your goals more realistic and therefore easier to achieve. These are the foundations of your long term goal. If you get these right, your medium and long term goals should follow.

Remember, keep your goals **SMART**. You can check off each one against the "smart-o-meter" as you write them, to ensure that each goal will be achievable for you. Your long and medium term goals do not have to fulfil these requirements, but it is really important that your short term goals do. Is it:

Specific?

Measurable?

Agreed?

Realistic?

Time-scaled?

My long term goals

Record your long term goals.

My medium term goals

Record your medium term goals. This should be the bridge between your short and long term goals, so link them if you can.

My short term goals

Use this space to record your short term goals.

" A goal without a plan is just a wish"

Antoine de Saint-Exupery

Things keeping me in my Comfort Zone

List the things that are keeping you in your Comfort Zone. Next to each, think of a strategy that you can use to move you forward. Draw on all your resources of vision, positive thinking, challenging negative beliefs, goal setting, safety netting, time management, team building and reward.

Things keeping me in my Comfort Zone	Strategies for moving forward

"Habit is habit and not to be flung out of the window by any man, but coaxed downstairs one step at a time"

Mark Twain

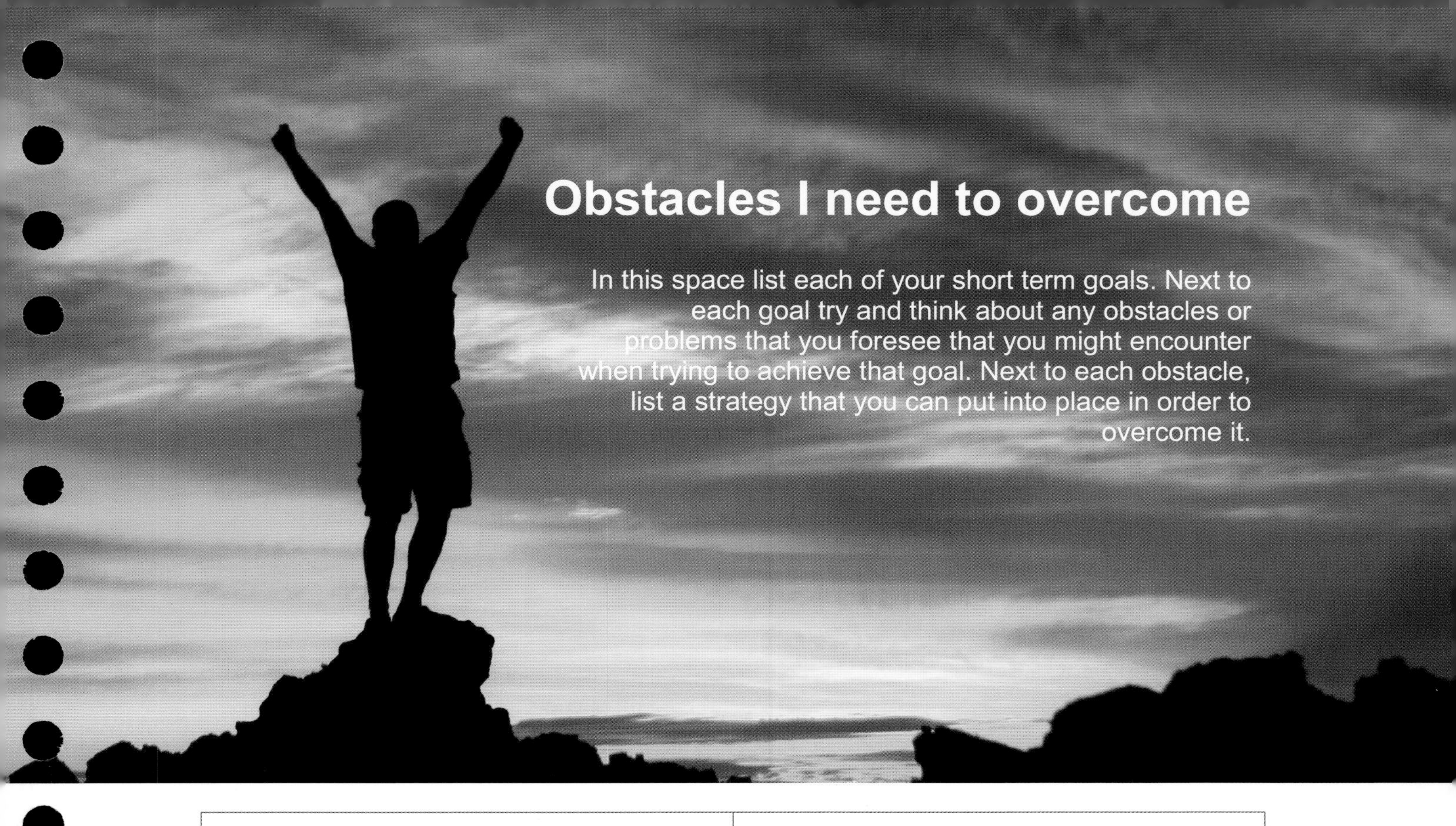

Obstacles I need to overcome

In this space list each of your short term goals. Next to each goal try and think about any obstacles or problems that you foresee that you might encounter when trying to achieve that goal. Next to each obstacle, list a strategy that you can put into place in order to overcome it.

Obstacles I need to overcome	Strategies

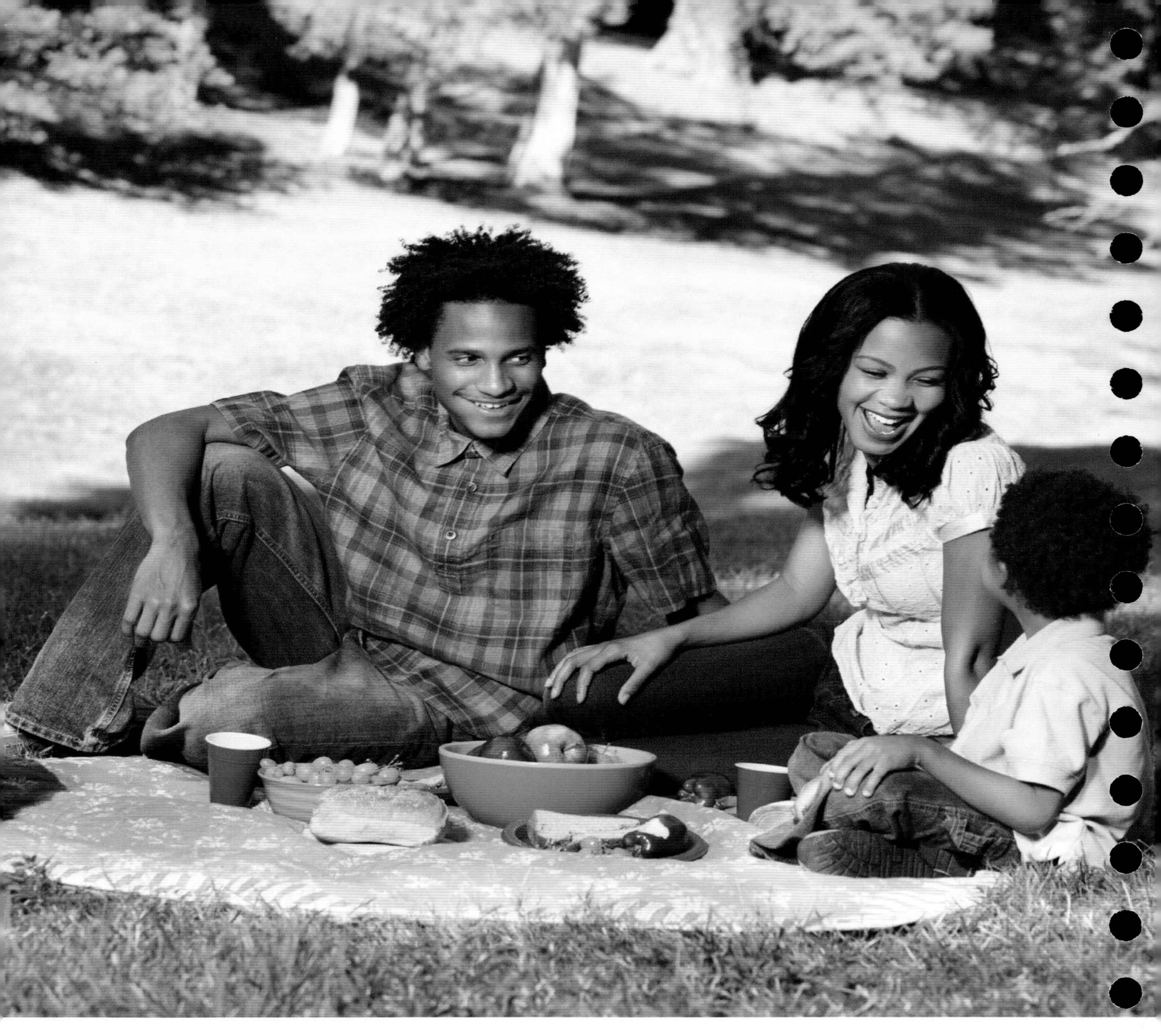

Your Weekly Planner

I have included an empty Weekly Planner on the page overleaf. You can use this to help you plan yours and your family's week. See pages 125-126 for ideas on how to fill it in using colour coding.

If you find that there is not enough room on the plan, you can use the idea of "roles and goals" to make your plan and then transfer your plan to a diary. You can also download a copy of the Weekly Planner from the web site accompanying the book on www.healthcompass.co.uk .

You don't have to use the same roles that I have used on page 126. This is just a guide.

I find that a diary which shows a whole week across two pages the best.

Weekly planner		Weekly Activity Planner Appointments and Commitments						
Roles	Goals	Monday	Tuesday	Wednesday	Thursday	Friday	Saturday	Sunday
		8am	8am	8am	8am	8am	8am	8am
		9	9	9	9	9	9	9
		10	10	10	10	10	10	10
		11	11	11	11	11	11	11
		12	12	12	12	12	12	12
		1pm	1pm	1pm	1pm	1pm	1pm	1pm
		2	2	2	2	2	2	2
		3	3	3	3	3	3	3
		4	4	4	4	4	4	4
		5	5	5	5	5	5	5
		6	6	6	6	6	6	6
		7	7	7	7	7	7	7
		8pm	8pm	8pm	8pm	8pm	8pm	8pm
		9	9	9	9	9	9	9
		10	10	10	10	10	10	10

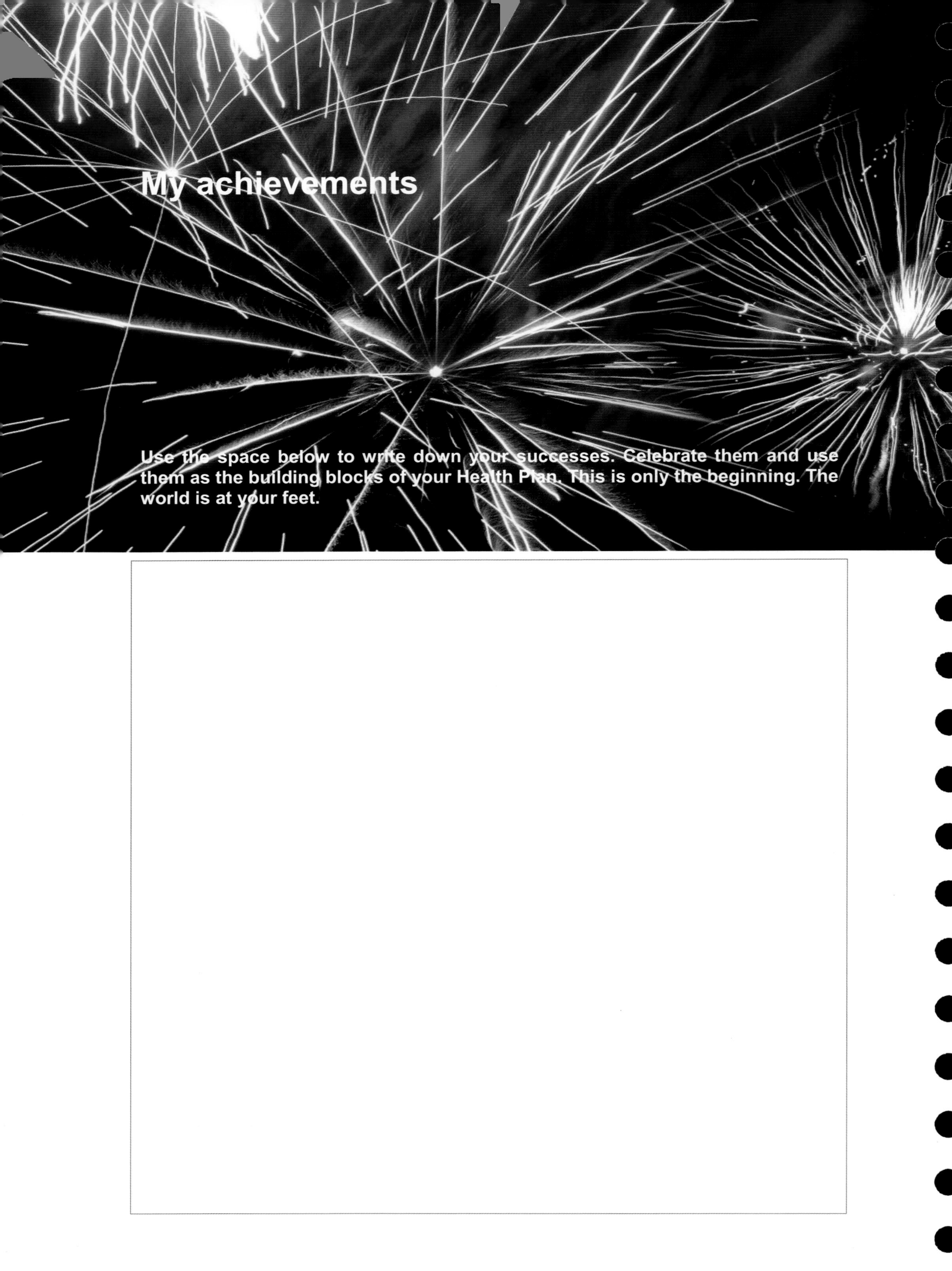

My achievements

Use the space below to write down your successes. Celebrate them and use them as the building blocks of your Health Plan. This is only the beginning. The world is at your feet.

My goal evaluation

If you have struggled or have not been successful in your attempt at a particular goal, make a note of why you did not succeed and what you will do in subsequent attempts to improve your chances of success.

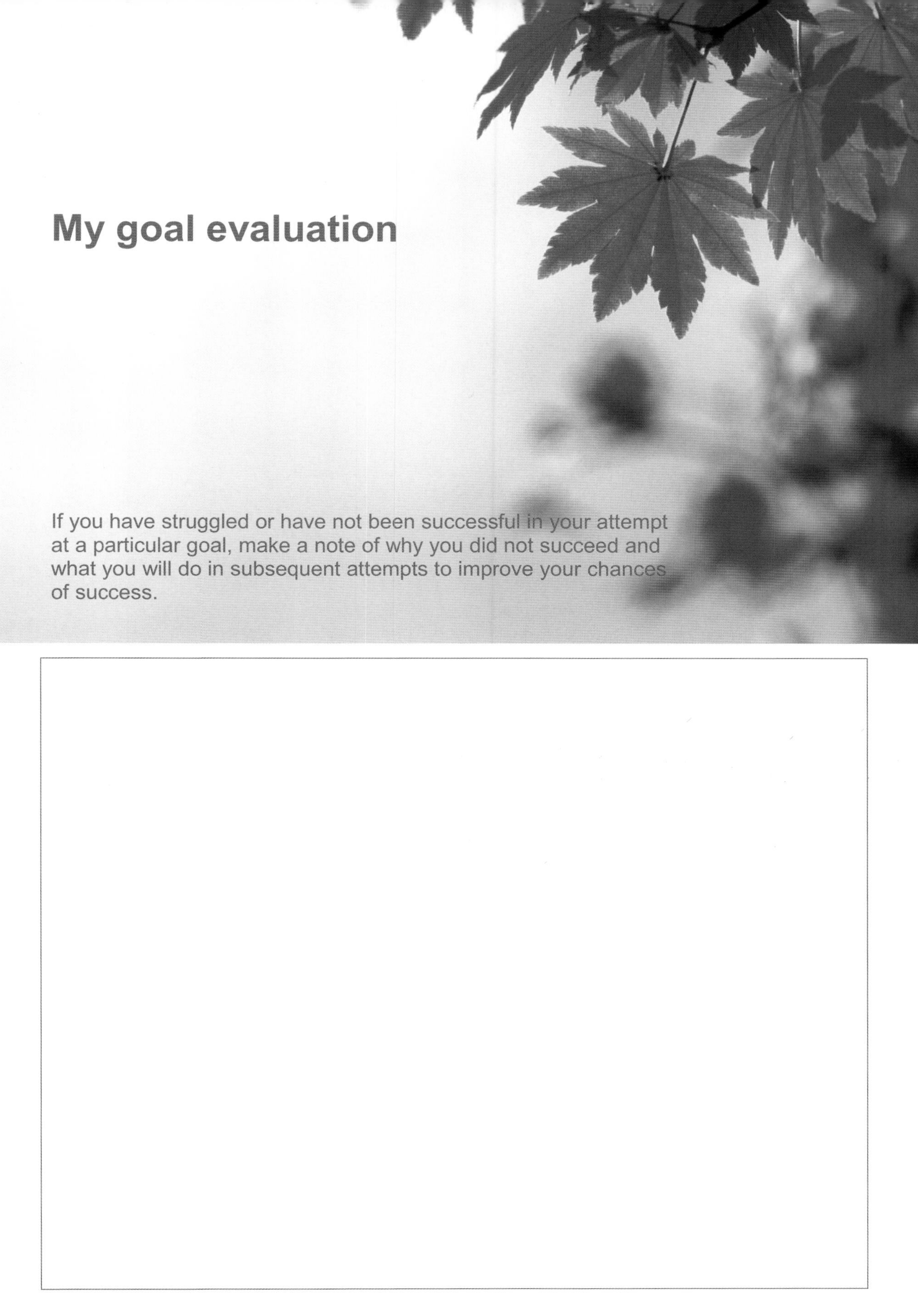

"If you have made mistakes, even serious ones, there is always another chance for you. What we call failure is not the falling down, but the staying down"

Mary Pickford

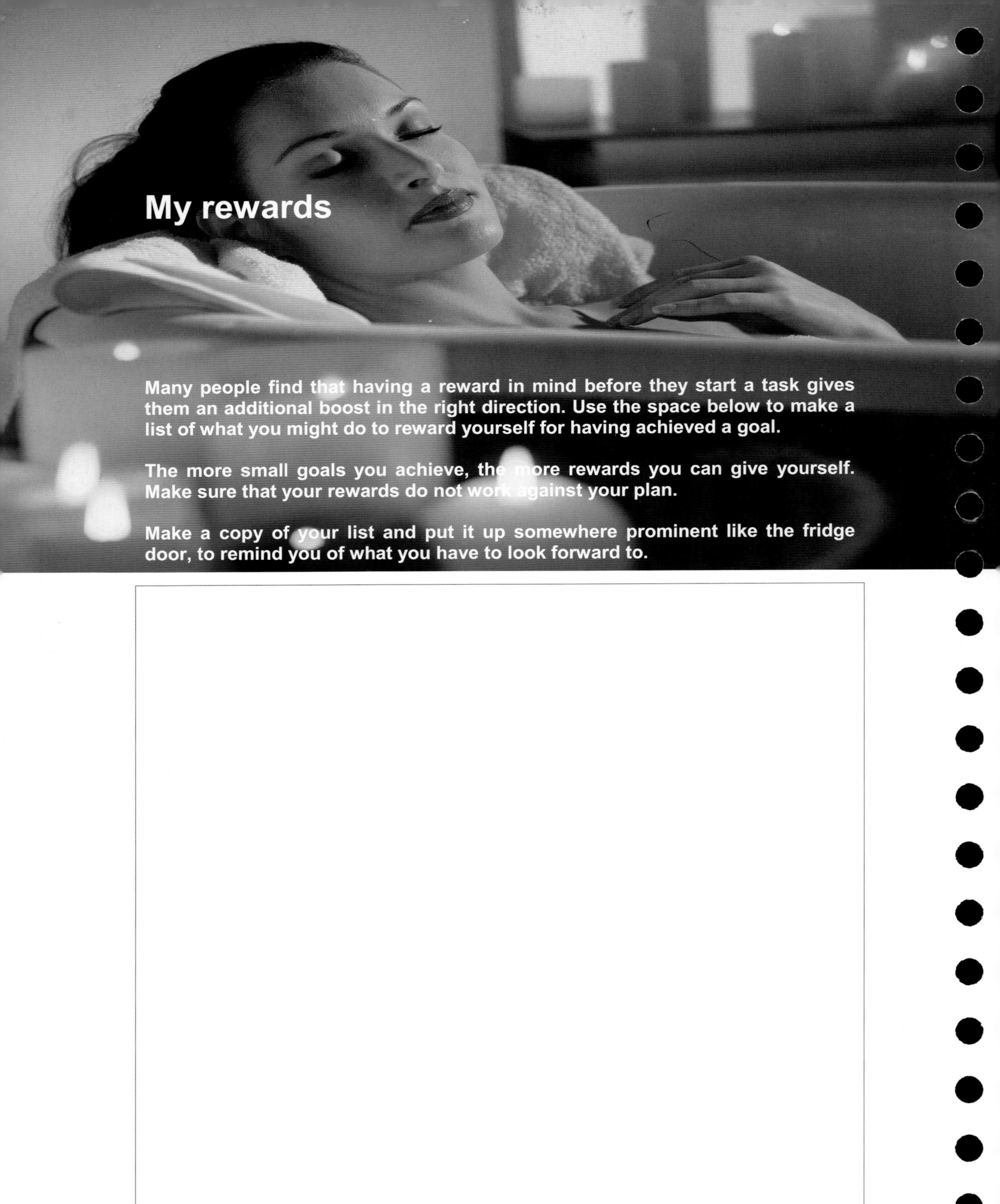

My rewards

Many people find that having a reward in mind before they start a task gives them an additional boost in the right direction. Use the space below to make a list of what you might do to reward yourself for having achieved a goal.

The more small goals you achieve, the more rewards you can give yourself. Make sure that your rewards do not work against your plan.

Make a copy of your list and put it up somewhere prominent like the fridge door, to remind you of what you have to look forward to.

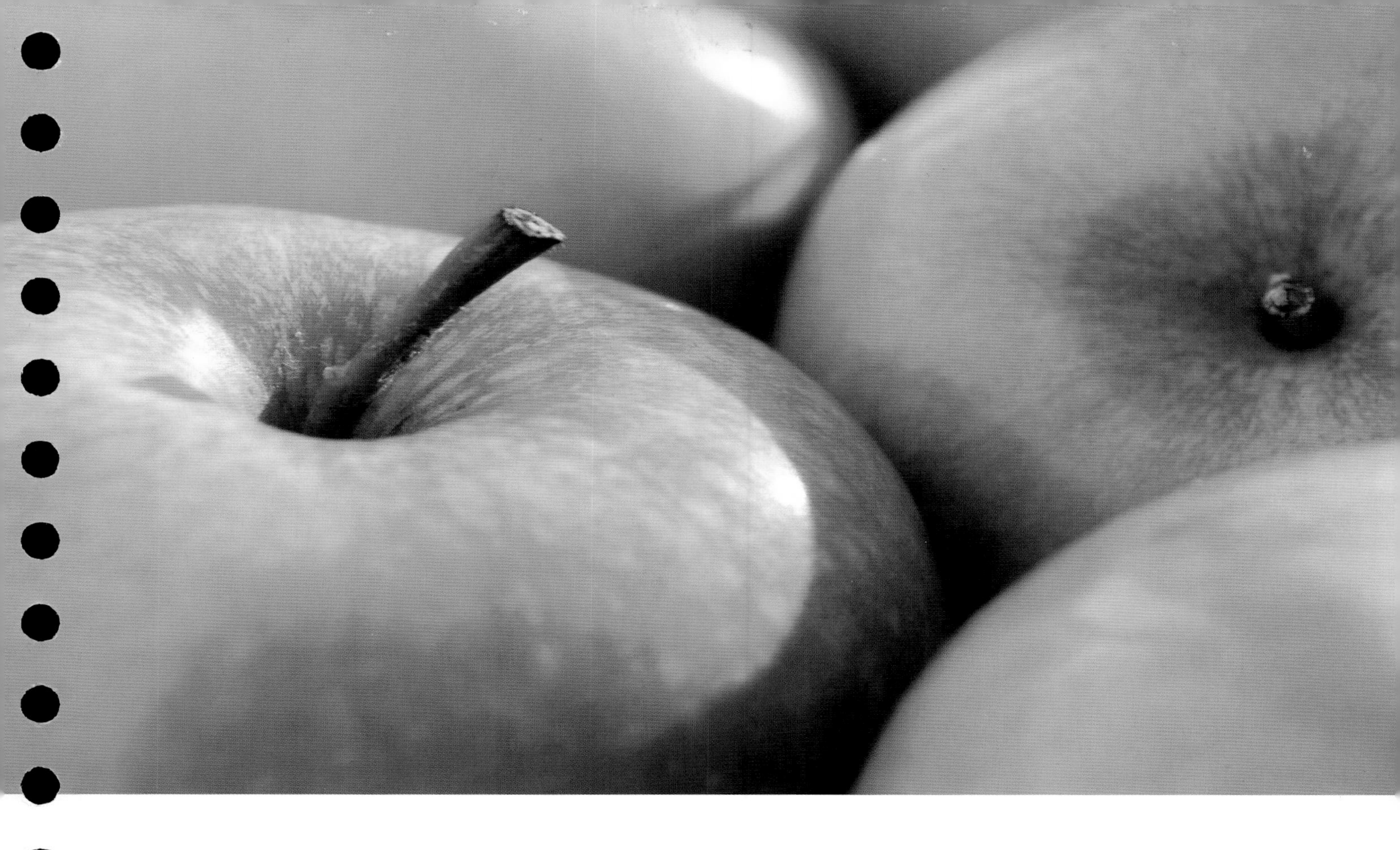

Congratulations

You have everything you need to lead you to great things.

Celebrate your successes and use the confidence this brings you as a boost for new or bigger goals. Look forward to what you can achieve. Plan how you will get there. Congratulate yourself when you do. Look back and see how far you have come.

Live your life the way you want to live it, to the best of your ability. Make your mark. Show others how it can be done.

It's your life; you have one chance at it

Make it work for you

You can do it

Contacts (Are we nearly there yet?)

Contact	Telephone	Web address
Alcohol Concern	0207 264 0510	www.alcoholconcern.org.uk
Alcoholics Anonymous	0845 769 7555	www.alcoholics-anonymous.org.uk
NHS Smoking pregnancy helpline	0800 169 9169	
NHS Smoking helpline	0800 169 0169	
Quit line	0800 00 22 00	
Nice guidance on NRT	0870 1555 455 ref N0084	
British Complementary Medical Association	0845 345 5977	www.bcma.co.uk
Institute for Complementary Med.	020 7237 5165	www.icmedicine.co.uk
The Calvert Trust	01598 763 221	www.calvert-trust.org.uk
The Health Compass		www.healthcompass.co.uk
Orlistat weight loss programme		www.xenicalmap.co.uk
Sibutramine weight loss programme (free)		www.changeforlifeonline.com
British Obesity Services Patient's Association. Information on weight loss surgery		www.bospa.org
Weight loss surgery		www.patient.co.uk/showdoc/40025123
National Cycle Scheme		www.cyclescheme.co.uk
Geo-caching		www.geocache.co.uk
Letterboxing		www.letterboxingondartmoor.co.uk

Find the sport for you	www.sportengland.org/index/get_active/find_the_sport_for_you.htm
Walk in a group	www.whi.org.uk
National Cycling networks	www.bikeforall.net
Swimming regimes to build fitness, for all levels	www.swim4fitness.com
Swimathon sponsored event	www.swimathon.org
National women's running organisation-local groups and events	www.womensrunningnetwork.co.uk
British Military Fitness groups.	www.britmilfit.com
Find a personal trainer	www.exerciseregister.org
Find sports facilities you can use if you have a disability	www.inclusivefitness.org
Find exercises you can do if you have a disability	www.ncpad.org
Walks with the ramblers association for those with disability	www.ramblers.org.uk/INFO/everyone/disability.html
Exercises for the very overweight	www.obesityservices.org
Sustrans, sustainable transport charity	www.sustrans.org.uk
The National Trust	www.nationaltrust.org.uk/volunteering/
Free government stop smoking plan and information	www.gosmokefree.co.uk
Free stop smoking plan and information	www.newash.org.uk
National Institute for Clinical Excellence information on Nicotine Replacement Therapy	www.nice.org.uk/page.aspx?o=30631
Jack Russell, Personal Development Coach, Inspirational speaker, Outdoor Specialist.	www.pdcinspiration.com

Sources of Information (Roadside rescue)

Gilmore J. BMI and Health Rep. Statistics. Canada 1999, 11 (1):31-43

Obesity. National Institute for Clinical Excellence. December 2006

Lightening the Load. Tackling Overweight and Obesity. Produced by the National Heart Forum in association with the Faculty of Public Health and the Department of Health

Dhurandher N.V. et al. Association of adenovirus infection with human obesity. Obesity Research. 1997, 5:464-469

Dhurandhar NV et al: Asssociation of adenovirus infection with human obesity. Obesity Research 5:464-469, 1997.

Taheri S: The link between short sleep duration and obesity. Arch. Dis. Child. 2006 Nov:91 (11): 881-4

So you want to lose weight for good. British Heart Foundation. 2006

Reducing your blood cholesterol. British Heart Foundation. 2007

Physical Activity and Your Heart. The British Heart Foundation 2005.

ACSM's Guidelines for Exercise Testing and Prescription

Four commonly used methods to increase physical activity: brief interventions in primary care, exercise referral schemes, pedometers and community based exercise programmes for walking and cycling. NICE March 2006

Randomised controlled trial of home-based walking programmes at and below current recommended levels of exercise in sedentary adults. Mark Tully et al. J. Epidemiol. Community Health, Sep 2007; 61: 778-783

Exercise in Pregnancy. Royal College of Obstetricians and Gynaecologists. Statement no. 4. January 2006

That's the Limit. Health Education Authority. London.1991

Alcohol Concern fact sheets. www.alcoholconcern.org.uk

Alcohol Consumption and Mortality: Modelling risks for men and women at different ages. Ian R White, Dan Altman, Kiran Nanchahal. BMJ. 2002; 325:191 (27 July)

Smoking and Your Heart. The British Heart Foundation. 2004

Giving Up For Life. Department of Health. 2002

Smoking Cessation-Bupropion and Nicotine Replacement therapy. National Institute for Health and Clinical Excellence. March 2002

Don't Tell The Bumblebee. Jack Russell. PDC Inspiration. 2006

The Seven Habits of Highly Effective People. Stephen R. Covey. 1989

"Be careful about reading health books. You may die of a misprint"
Mark Twain